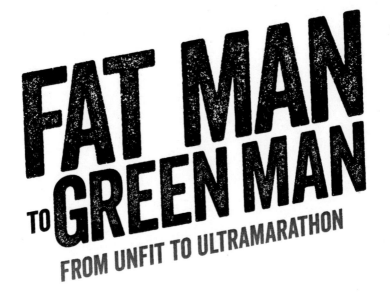

FAT MAN TO GREEN MAN

FROM UNFIT TO ULTRAMARATHON

IRA RAINEY

 BEARS

◆Tangent Books

This edition published 2014 by Tangent Books

Tangent Books
Unit 5.16 Paintworks
Bristol
BS4 3EH
0117 972 0645
www.tangentbooks.co.uk

ISBN 978-1-910089-01-9

This book is dedicated to
Remo Del-Greco
A friend and inspiration. Rest well.

Contents

Prologue

"If you have a body, you are an athlete." – **Bill Bowerman**

Sitting around in shorts basking in the warm Lanzarote sun was always going to be a preferable way to spend the final week of tapering after a number of months hard winter training in the UK. Whilst winding your mileage down to almost nothing before a big race is generally considered good practise, it also has the bizarre side-effect of making you feel extremely lethargic and convincing you that you've completely forgotten how to run. Quite how hundreds of miles and months of running could be mentally cancelled out by a few of days lying poolside with a paperback I'm not quite sure, but by midweek my legs felt distinctly wooden. I decided to try and shake the feeling by going out for a short jog around the resort, taking random left and right turns, heading off in the general direction of the coast in search of the sea. After a couple of miles, distracted by picturesque palm trees and gleaming white apartment buildings, I found myself in the centre of an exclusive gated complex where a group of leathery looking people were placing towels on sun loungers at eight o'clock in the morning. I stood around momentarily looking for a way down onto the paved promenade I could see outside but all the gates I approached were locked. As I ran around the numerous pools looking for an exit, to looks of concern and confusion from the leather people, I spotted a couple of security guards walking in my general direction – casually, yet with a distinct sense of purpose: nonchalant yet menacing. Looking around swiftly and with a mild sense of self-imposed panic I spy what looks like the lowest section of wall to enable my escape onto the footpath below and ploughed through the black volcanic gravel flowerbeds towards the drop. Despite not being the highest part of the perimeter it was still at least a six foot drop to freedom but looking back and seeing the secret apartment police closing in, I took a breath and threw myself off the wall with all the gentle abandon of a fugitive who didn't really want to hurt himself, and ran off towards the harbour at enough of a pace to put distance between me and the authorities without actually running too hard – I was after all supposed to be trying to rest for the week.

Further down the promenade and safe from arrest I stopped and sat on a set of steps leading down from the walkway to a small sandy beach, looking out over the Strait of La Bocaina towards Fuerteventura. I don't know why watching waves lap up against a shore makes you to pause and contemplate, maybe it's the hypnotic white noise of the water crashing down onto the beach and sliding back out again that lulls you into a trance, or maybe it's a simple realisation that unless you're a pretty strong swimmer you've escaped just about as far as you can and all you can do now is sit there and face up to what's going on inside your head.

The power of mobile internet (together with the European Union capping of roaming data rates) made the fact that I was over sixteen-hundred miles from home a total irrelevance to keeping in touch with the world, allowing me to do so as easily from the beach as if I was sat at home in Bristol. I skimmed through the inbox on my phone and spotted an unread email letting me know that somebody else had just donated some of their hard-earned cash through my online charity page. The notification emails had become more frequent in recent days as the event was drawing near, highlighting the charitable generosity of friends and family, work colleagues and even complete strangers. The one common thread tying them all together being me – an eternally delusional optimist with an impending challenge that was making even my most experienced running friends offer up their praise and admiration, whilst simultaneously shaking their heads in disbelief. I contemplated the messages of luck and goodwill that had been rolling in and who they are from. Words like *"awe"* and *"inspiration"* seemed to be being bandied around with far more frequency than I had seen before, certainly when people were talking about me anyway. Being a delusional optimist meant that a lack of self-confidence wasn't something I often experienced, but as I sat there looking out over the calm blue stretch of water a sudden wave of doubt washed over me – had I completely underestimated the whole thing? Had my pathological inability to see myself fail gone too far this time? For the first time in six months I sat and really thought about the upcoming weekend and whether I had actually taken on something that was just too big. Something that blind faith in yourself alone won't get you through. But this is what I do, time and again, whether I like it or not that is how my brain works. I jump into things with a reckless hopeful idealism and without fully thinking at all about the finer details until much closer to the time.

A friend of mine once told me after her triple heart bypass operation that she had learnt to *"not sweat the small stuff"* and I guess that's what I do, I don't sweat stuff, largely by just not really thinking about anything. That's all fine when the stuff you're not thinking about is only small but with just three days to go until I was due to run sixty miles over little more than a twenty-four hour period, I was really beginning to wonder if I should have maybe sweated it all a little bit more.

1. Stronger, Faster, Fatter

"Life is too short to have anything but delusional notions about yourself." – **Gene Simmons**

Sunday morning runs were often just as much about a social and a natter as they were about notching up miles and nobody liked to talk more than Phil. A long-time friend and considerably better runner than me, Phil Westlake and I would arrange to meet every Sunday without fail. If I ever had any thoughts of slacking off and staying in bed I knew they would be fruitless, as he tolerated no excuses. When it's below zero and lashing down with rain, training with somebody so committed – and there were times I thought he really should be – meant you just got out and did it whatever the weather. It was character building apparently, *"once you're wet, you're wet"* I was always told and you just can't argue with logic like that.

We'd normally head out around the lanes, parks and footpaths of Bristol and the surrounding area for about an hour or two, pounding out loosely planned routes generally devised long before GPS or online mapping. In between the weekly catch-up I would often be regaled with recycled anecdotes of races past. Like the time his long-suffering wife Anita was beaten in a sprint finish by Rupert the Bear, or the race in Eastville Park where a guy turned up late and raced in his work trousers and shirt. There were many stories to tell and over the years I'd heard them all – countless times. But as a true friend and good listener I never let that be known, just nodding and agreeing in the right places seemed the proper thing to do. Sometimes I might fill in some minor detail he couldn't recall but only to expedite the tale, although he never noticed.

Today though was a different conversation. Today it was all about a book he'd read recently about a runner who ran ultramarathons, whatever they were. I could tell from the raised tone and excited inflection of his voice as he was talking that he was clearly quite taken aback by what he'd read. *"And he carried on running through the night scoffing pizza and cheesecake he'd had delivered to him whilst he was out running!"* Phil exclaimed. It was December 2010 and on the strength of that statement alone I made sure *Ultramarathon Man* by Dean Karnazes was mentioned in my letter to Santa. I'd never heard of Karnazes before and I wasn't entirely sure what an ultramarathon was but it sounded like it was worth a read. From the moment I picked up the book on Christmas Day I became engrossed in tales of epic challenges such as the Western States 100 and the Badwater Ultramarathon. Despite my almost remedial reading speed and the fact that I spent a large part of the day gorging on seasonal fare followed by settling down to the obligatory Doctor Who Christmas special, I had finished it cover to cover by Boxing Day. It was incredible reading. Karnazes was some kind of running savant who tucked his kids up in bed and then went out and ran huge distances through the night before rocking up to work the next morning. He ran in races hundreds of miles long, across snow and through deserts and wrote about it all in a very accessible way.

Earlier that year I had watched a BBC documentary about the comedian Eddie Izzard who ran forty-three marathons in fifty-one days for Sport Relief, despite having never really run before. It was a truly remarkable undertaking that raised over a million pounds for charity, but this ultrarunning lark Karnazes wrote about was something else again, raising the whole thing to another level. Take the Badwater Ultramarathon for example. Billed as the world's toughest foot race, it is 135 miles long and runs through Death Valley,

California – officially the hottest place on Earth – in the height of summer. To top that off it also finishes with a climb of 8360 feet just to make it a bit more interesting. Karnazes won this race in 2004 – aged forty-one – in a time of 27 hours, 22 minutes and 48 seconds. But there's no big prize money on offer at Badwater. Other than a t-shirt for finishing, the only award is a paltry commemorative belt buckle – which, as shiny and lovely as it is, doesn't even come with a belt attached – and even that requires a sub forty-eight hour finish. The book opened my eyes to a world of running that I knew nothing about. It was one full of insanely long races completed by runners with otherworldly levels of stamina and fitness. Distance running superheroes, only without the capes and masks.

I was no stranger to running, I'd been plugging away at it for a number of years, but I'd certainly never really been what you would term an athlete, nor had I ever entertained the slightest notion that I could tackle the Herculean challenges guys like Karnazes completed with their eyes closed. Despite the fact that I loved Marvel comics when I was a kid and so wanted to be superhuman, as much as I hoped and dreamed, it was very apparent from an early age that I had no fantastic powers. Like many young comic fans I could often be found running around the garden with one of my mum's old curtains tied around my neck thinking I could fly, although coincidentally only as far as I could jump. That kind of delusion was not uncommon for me when I was young and although I never actually believed myself to have mutant powers or to have been born on a far off planet, I did know that I was different to everybody else.

I grew up in the suburbs of Bristol, in a happy family where my parents weren't violent, didn't drink excessively and nobody really got sick. It was all quite twee and uneventful. In fact you could've said we were almost middle class if it wasn't for the free school dinners, second-hand school uniform and a 10p slot meter for the electric. I was always a quiet and oblivious child, who lacked many real friends. I had siblings and we got on OK, but my brother was always too young to be on my level and my older sister was, well, a girl.

It's not that I wasn't friendly with other kids, I tried to be, but generally their parents thought I was unbalanced and a bad influence. I knew I wasn't unhinged; I was just different, because you see I was a robot. An amazingly realistic robot I had to admit, in fact so realistic even I'd always be amazed at the sight of my own blood. My skin was soft to touch, my hair was big and even from an early age I appeared to be gaining a tubby persuasion – probably part of the reason I couldn't fly I thought. Robots weren't exactly commonplace in Bristol in the 1970s; in fact the only other robot I knew of at the time was my only real friend Hugo, who like me was convinced of his own mechanical status. Secretly though I knew he was an imposter, mostly because he had bandy legs and all kids know nobody can bend metal. But I had to humour him, as my mum said he was unbalanced.

I never really told anyone about me being a robot, mostly because as my parents never mentioned it I guessed it must have been highly classified. To complicate matters further I wasn't very magnetic, I couldn't spin my head right around and even though I did try drinking motor oil once it only made me ill. I figured it was probably the wrong viscosity for the time of year. I was confused. Was I a robot or not? I was convinced I was but I didn't exactly fit the mould. Then – out of the blue – came the explanation I so desperately needed. On my fifth birthday, September 12th 1974, I received a present that explained everything. It wasn't a book or a toy but simply the permission to stay up late and watch television. There, on HTV at seven-thirty that fateful Wednesday evening I was presented with my answer: The Six Million Dollar Man. *"Steve Austin, a man barely alive. Gentleman, we can rebuild him. We have the technology; we have the capability to make the world's first bionic man. Steve Austin will be that man, whether he likes it or not. Better than he was before, better, stronger, faster."*

All of a sudden everything was clear, that was it, I wasn't a robot at all – I was bionic. I was Ira Austin, Steve Rainey, Ira Lee Majors; I was the two and a half million pound* bionic Bristolian boy. I sprinted out of the house on a new found lease of atomic energy and ran at extreme speeds around our cul-de-sac until I had an asthma attack and passed out outside the library. As I came around tucked up in bed, my mum tried to explain to me the dangers of watching science fiction when you're not old enough to realise it isn't real, but I pretended not to hear, which was quite a difficult task with bionic hearing.

Despite my bionic implants I was never sporty or particularly active at school and I certainly never ran. I suffered from a touch of asthma at the time and whenever cross country came around I was often the one with a note from my mum excusing me from joining in. I always assumed this was just to help keep my cover, as if I ran around the school field at 60mph I could've been rumbled. This generally worked well for me, other than the time I tried jumping over the racks in the bike shed while everyone else was playing football. Trying to keep it steady so as to not jump too high and attract attention, I caught my foot on a snapped-off upright stand, fell and gashed my right knee wide open. I ruined a perfectly good pair of second-hand school trousers and ended up being carried by Mr Shannon, our French teacher, to his car and then into A&E at Frenchay Hospital where I was graced with five stitches. However that was in the early 1980s before health and safety had been invented, so nobody really got into any trouble.

It was as I moved through secondary school that I began to suspect that my bionics might not be as real as I'd envisaged. What

---

* Great exchange rates back in September 1974 – $2.3175 to the pound.

else could explain having to wear National Health glasses and coming last in almost every athletics event I took part in? All of a sudden growing up sucked. Without any form of robotic or bionic assistance I was just a normal chubby kid with big hair who was crap at sport. So there and then I decided to do something about it – I gave up. I gave up on sport and generally being outside, becoming a fully-fledged computer nerd instead. The only exercise I entertained through most of the mid-1980s was waggling a Quickshot joystick to destruction whilst playing Daley Thompson's Decathlon on the Commodore 64. My only exposure to real sport through those indoor years was the spectacle that was Saturday afternoon wrestling on World of Sport with Dickie Davies. A world where men were called Shirley, twenty stone was considered a lightweight and the term athlete was stretching it about as far as the wrestlers' leotards. Between that and the Sunday afternoon darts quiz Bullseye, I figured I had the full spectrum of sport covered. They were dark years.

It wasn't until many years later, at the start of the new millennium, that I actually bought myself a pair of trainers and started to run. I had decided, out of the blue, to take on the Bristol Half Marathon after seeing it advertised in the Bristol Evening Post, thinking it sounded like a bit of fun. Hindsight is a wonderful thing and I can see now that I had absolutely no idea what I was doing and no clue as to what I was letting myself in for. Fun is very definitely a misguided term when it comes to running 13.1 miles. However, despite all the odds and just six weeks of half-hearted and ill-considered training around the hilly streets of Totterdown, I somehow managed to finish in 2 hours 6 minutes. The distinct lack of preparation however, coupled with the fact that somebody twice my size stood on my foot as I was collecting my medal, made the mile walk back home take almost half as long as the previous 13.1. It also consigned me to taking the lift up one floor at work for the best part of two weeks. The whole experience put me right off running. I wasn't a runner; my big-boned non-bionic frame just wasn't built for it. No, I just liked a challenge and now it was accomplished I could happily slide back into my previous sloth-like existence, and that is exactly what I did for a good few years, whilst eating and drinking aplenty. I didn't miss running at all, why would I? It was bloody hard work and it wasn't like I was ever going to win anything for my efforts. No, with the half marathon box ticked I threw my trainers into the back of the cupboard and forgot all about them for a number of years. That was until the day I caught sight of myself in a mirror and realised that I had started to resemble one of my wrestling heroes of yesteryear. I may not have been called Shirley nor did I own a leotard, but I was certainly starting to sport a stomach that would firmly test the stretchability of one. Not being a gym or a diet kind of guy I fished around in the back of the cupboard and pulled out my cobweb-laced trainers and started running again in a bid to try and manage my weight and fitness. That was 2002 and for some inexplicable reason, I kind of stuck with it, running a few miles here and there although nothing very serious. A few years later, after changing jobs and being unable to plod around during my lunch hour, following a recommendation from Phil I semi-reluctantly joined my local running club, Bitton Road Runners. Being a miserable bastard at heart, going running with a group of strangers didn't initially hold any appeal whatsoever. I wasn't really interested in the social or friendship element of being part of a club; I just wanted more motivation to keep running, so I gave it a go. In the end, despite my best curmudgeonly efforts, joining Bitton turned out to have the single biggest impact on my running to date. I met a whole new group of perfectly normal like-minded people of all abilities; I ran more, trained better and raced harder. Over the years that followed I ran in countless 5K and 10K races, fifteen half marathons and completed three marathons. I even actually enjoyed some of them. I had now become a proper runner.

spirits, I figured I was fine. I always saw it more as habitual drinking; I did it because I did it yesterday, or because that's just what I did on a Friday. Whatever the label or excuse, the end result is much the same to your health. If the first place you go after a hard track session is the off licence to grab a six pack as a reward for running hard, you're not really taking your training very seriously. When you walk into a supermarket and your seven-year-old son asks you if we're here just to buy beer again, I think it's fair to say that you're probably in that aisle a little bit more often than you should be. The easy solution is just not to take your kids shopping but that doesn't really address the core issue. Spells of eating and drinking to excess interspersed with short bouts of trying to lose weight was more or less the loop I'd been stuck on for as long as I could remember.

Weight had always been an issue for me as an adult and it had never completely been under control. I used to think that throughout my many years of running, I had generally been slim and fit with a couple of spells of being overweight and unfit, but when I sat back and thought about it I could see that actually it had largely been the other way around. I always liked to believe that I could carry off a few extra pounds as I stood pretty tall at six feet, although talking to people about it honestly, apparently I was wrong. At my peak weight I'd squeezed seventeen and a half stone into the trousers of denial, and at my lightest point had fleetingly dropped to a touch over fourteen stone. Neither end of the scale was going to break any kind of obesity record or get me on any kind of voyeuristic Channel 4 show but it was certainly far from an ideal place to be, especially if you're trying to be athletic. Running plenty of miles when you're heavy can still lead to improvements in fitness. A study published in the *European Heart Journal* in 2012 highlighted the fact that you can in fact be fat and fit. Examining data on over 43,000 people researchers determined that being overweight or obese did not necessarily increase your chance of dying from heart disease or cancer, providing you were metabolically fit. From a running perspective you would obviously benefit from not carrying extra weight around with you but you would get used to it and your muscles would build in strength to cope with the demand. You'd be slower than you could be but you'd still be running. It's for this very reason that I came to be awarded the nickname of Bumblebee.

In 2009 scientists at Oxford University's Department of Zoology used a wind-tunnel, smoke and high-speed cameras to study the flight of the humble bumble, *Bombus terrestris*. What they found was a creature that was incredibly inefficient – aerodynamically speaking – but that against all odds managed to fly using brute force rather than wing-flapping finesse. Here was the basis of my nickname, not because of a love of honey, or a penchant for stripy black and yellow shirts, but apparently because although I could run a bit, I was actually so fat I didn't look like I should be able to. If you would like to pause reading this book for a second and look up the phrase *'backhanded compliment'* in the nearest dictionary, I think you will find this as an example.

At my heaviest point I was squarely classified as obese - a whole bracket more than just overweight. I've always thought that it's not a very nice looking word, obese. Maybe that's the point, it's not meant to be. As an adjective it's certainly far from the most offensive thing a person could be characterised as but it's certainly not a word that has a hugely positive purpose in life. It's just got nothing going for it – it's not even going to land you a high score in Scrabble. Unfortunately for me however it was factually accurate in a descriptive sense. I remember when I was about ten years old once asking my mum if my dad's extra-large trousers would fit me when I was a grown-up and they both just laughed. Looking back now I don't know if that was just because they found my juvenile naivety humorous and endearing, or if it was actually nervous laughter attempting to mask the inevitable truth of beef dripping and genetics from a child. As a kid I always thought that middle-aged spread was something my dad had in his sandwiches, but now I realise it had been in mine all along too. Maybe I should've stuck with the free school dinners.

It was summer 2012 and it was all a bit out of control really. My forty-third birthday was fast approaching making it pretty evident that I wasn't getting any younger and I most certainly wasn't getting any slimmer. I really wanted to do something about it although in truth I was just too lazy to put the effort in or make any sacrifices to look after my own body. Part of being delusional means that you often think that everything will be just fine, regardless of your actions. Then one day late in July I was called into an ad-hoc meeting at work with the rest of our small team by my boss, Remo. He'd been off for a few days and had just popped into the office for a quick meeting to update us all with some news. Without any drama or self-pity he sat there and calmly told us that he had been diagnosed with stage four oesophageal cancer and had been given six to nine months to live. It was absolutely devastating news that nobody had seen coming. Here was a seemingly fit and healthy guy in his fifties with everything going for him. He was a husband, a father of five and a friend. I sat next to him every day and we always enjoyed a good bit of banter and fun amongst the work. The news absolutely hit me for six, not just the severity of it but the extremely stoic way with which he handled it all. He left and we all held it together in the office for the next couple of hours in a typically British way, mostly I think still in shock. As I drove home tears began to flow uncontrollably and by the time I got there and broke the news to my wife I was a wreck. As a child whenever I clashed with my mum and told her something just wasn't fair, she always stopped the argument in its tracks with a simple *"Life's not fair"*. That day I realised she was right.

Up until that point I had been extremely lucky in my life and, other than my grandparents, I hadn't suffered any particularly close personal losses or tragedies. I know that people die every day, people deal with loss and the world carries on regardless, but when it is so tragic and so close it really does make you stop and think about your own life and what you're doing with it. Life can be so brief and it should be lived to the full and with my slacker attitude I realised I wasn't exactly giving myself the best chance of doing that. Whilst you never know what your body has genetically scheduled for you, the very least you can do, the very least you owe yourself and those around you, is to stay in as good health as possible so as to maximise your chances of longevity. Isn't that just sensible?

Over the next few days I decided that I really had to take some decisive action. I wanted to tackle my age-old bad habits for good, lose some serious weight and coerce myself into taking my health and fitness much more seriously. Running would be key to this, that much I knew, but running what? Having taken on the half marathon distance so many times, even whilst being properly fat, I knew that wouldn't do it, nor being honest would a marathon – I'd been there done that and got several t-shirts (although none that really fitted). That's when Karnazes' superhuman tales of extreme distances and eating on the move flashed back through my mind. We were about the same age, were we so different? Well obviously yes, I hadn't run across America, but hey, I liked running and I loved eating – both things an ultramarathon dictates you to do quite a lot of – it sounded like my kind of event. Maybe that was the answer – a massive mileage challenge. But wasn't it just the runner's equivalent of buying a convertible and trying to cop off with someone half their age – a mid-life crisis with trainers and power gels? It certainly had a ring of trying to prove oneself to it, proving that despite the beer belly and the balding crown, there was life in these old bionic legs yet.

Maybe just as OSI* rebuilt Steve Austin I too could be rebuilt into something better, something stronger, faster and slightly less fat – maybe even slim for once in my life. I liked the idea; it was a positive one, a call to action, a challenge, but which ultra should I sign up for? The Western States 100 maybe? How about Badwater? I could take on Karnazes at his own game. I don't know though, they both seemed such long way to go to just get a belt buckle, and I'm not sure it would even fit on my £3 reversible canvas belt from Matalan.

No, I needed something closer to home and perhaps a tad shorter and cooler than a 135 mile climb through Death Valley. That's when I remembered a conversation I'd had with Bill Graham, one of the coaches at Bitton Road Runners, about an event he'd ran earlier in the year. It was a race that looped all the way around Bristol following a footpath called the Community Forest Path. At around forty-six miles in length it certainly fell under the classification of an ultramarathon and being in Bristol meant I could sleep in my own bed at both ends of the day – providing I finished before the day was up. It sounded ideal, other than the having to run forty-six miles bit. If anything was going to make me start taking my weight and running more seriously it was the thought of having to slog my fat ass around the woods of Bristol from dawn till dusk at the tail end of winter.

So that was it, without hesitation; without really thinking it through; and without explaining to my wife that I would be spending most of the winter out running, the challenge was on – I was going to tackle The Green Man Ultra. I loaded up the website and completed the entry form, pausing momentarily at the £45 entry fee – almost one pound per mile – was that the price of redemption? Click,

---

* The Office of Scientific Intelligence was the secret government organisation who were responsible for sticking the batteries into Steve Austin and sending him on all manner of jobs.

submit, done. There was no going back now. The fat man would take on the Green Man, face-to-face in a personal battle of strength, determination and mud. Only one could win but who would it be? As I put my wallet back away in my pocket and slowly closed the lid of my laptop, I quietly hoped it wasn't going to be the other guy.

2. Of Woodwose and Wistman

"The woods are lovely dark and deep,
but I have promises to keep,
and miles to go before I sleep,
and miles to go before I sleep." – **Robert Frost**

Not being Bear Grylls, Little Red Riding Hood, or a closet lumberjack, I'd not tended to spend a huge chunk of my life in the woods. Past climbing trees as a child, I never felt the need or inclination to visit more often. Woods are always portrayed as dark and dingy places where, as children are often told, bears collectively eat picnics on a daily basis. If I had grown up in the American Midwest then I'm sure I would have been taken into the wilderness as a boy and taught how to hunt and kill by my father, as he was by his – taught how to fire a gun; how to be self-sufficient in the wild; and how to stitch up my own wounds like a junior John Rambo. Growing up in seventies suburban Bristol however the closest I got to learning any woodland skills was climbing trees whilst scrumping* and shooting at empty baked bean tins with my dad's air rifle. I did fleetingly have a chance of gaining an adventure badge in the Boys' Brigade but not before I was thrown out for failing to attend church services (apparently quite important for members of a Christian youth organisation). So exactly what grounding or qualifications I thought I had to take on a forty-six mile run through Bristol's distributed woodland I'm not quite sure. To complicate matters further the Community Forest

---

* Scrumping – to climb somebody else's apple tree and try to make off with as much fruit as you can before being shot at or caught. Good harmless crime for boys.

Path isn't exactly a footpath as a townie like me might think. To me a footpath is something that is designed for walking on, running if you're feeling sporty, but it's a pathway marked out and more importantly, surfaced ready for its sole purpose – ideally in slabs or tarmac. This however was an off-road event, also commonly known as multi-terrain – multi in this sense meaning both wet and muddy. Just when you thought it couldn't get any worse, it turned out the race route wasn't even really marked out – you had to navigate it all yourself following the forest path signs and using a good old-fashioned paper map. If you got lost, that was your problem. There were a handful of checkpoints along the way to check your progress and ensure you didn't keel over in a ditch and get forgotten about but you still had to find those. Despite being an optimist, even I had started to realise this race was going to be a big undertaking. However just like the very first half marathon I ran, it was a challenge and if other mere mortals could achieve it then so could I. Instead of the usual plodding up and down the Bristol to Bath cycletrack, this would take lots of off-road training, plenty of research of the route, and more importantly significant weight loss and a huge improvement in my fitness. It was clear this challenge wasn't going to be achieved with any old half-hearted attempt, which was entirely my plan.

The burning question though was who is the Green Man and why was he organising a race around Bristol in the first place? When I think of green men my mind immediately jumps back to my childhood, reading comics and watching trashy TV and I see Lou Ferrigno as The Incredible Hulk, getting all angry and throwing foam boulders around after losing another shirt (yet keeping his jeans). But I was pretty sure this race was nothing to do with him, Hulk was always much more of a smasher than a runner. Throw Bristol into the mental search engine though and the next person who pops up is Dave Prowse – The Green Cross Man.

Probably best known as the body of Darth Vader in the original Star Wars trilogy, Prowse was also a Bristolian seventies safety superhero, educating a whole generation of children on how to cross the road without being mown down by a speeding Austin Allegro, foolishly mixing cross-ply and radial tyres on the same axle. As part of a series of public information films a costumed Prowse would use his teleportation device to suddenly pop up on the roadside saving kids in the nick of time from certain Cortina doom before explaining the Green Cross Code to them and warning that he won't always be there when they crossed the road. Obviously being an avid superhero fan I loved the films, mostly as they proved you could be superhuman and broadly Bristolian at the same time – something Marvel comics never really portrayed. Was Prowse the green man in question?

Despite having his West Country Darth Vader dialogue overdubbed by James Earl Jones in the films, Prowse toured science fiction conventions talking about his time as part of the Star Wars universe. However, it had been widely reported that he had fallen out with George Lucas a number of times over the years and was now banned from official events. Whether that was true or not I didn't know but if so did he really need money so badly that he had to resort to playing on his seventies television fame and putting on a foot race around his home town? Maybe that's why it was all off-road – to keep everyone safe from traffic. Looking at the event details closer I couldn't find anything mentioning either Prowse or the Green Cross Code anywhere in the race information or on the website. Maybe he was actually fine for money after all and I had the wrong green man.

However after a bit more digging around it appeared I was actually (extremely tenuously) onto something, not with the Green Cross Code, but with Prowse's other alter ego, the Dark Lord of the Sith himself – Mr Vader. In Star Wars, Darth Vader is a master of using and manipulating the mystical power known as the Force. Lucas often described the Force as synonymous with a universal *'life force'* – an energy field created by all living things that was utilised by the powers of good and evil. Whilst this makes for the core of a great science fiction tale, like many film plot ideas it's certainly not a new one. The concept of some form of metaphysical power that pervades through all living things goes back thousands of years and is littered throughout history, both religious and secular. The Green Man, it turned out, was another manifestation of that same basic idea – a mystical life-giving force interweaved through the seasonal cycles of the woodland. He is everywhere, representing life, death and rebirth in the vegetative world. Steeped in myth and folklore, the Green Man can often be found watching over us as a decorative architectural ornament on churches and other buildings all around the world. He is commonly found as a carved wooden or stone face surrounded by, made up of, and sprouting leaves and other foliage. Ironically the National Cathedral in Washington DC actually has a stone Darth Vader head on its Northwest Tower – I wonder if Prowse gets a royalty for that?

The rather boring fact was that the Green Man Ultra was simply so named because of the giant carved stone head of a Green Man in the grounds of the Ashton Court mansion house in Bristol. Located in the red deer enclosure, the head marked the start and finish of a circumnavigation of the Community Forest Path known as the Green Man Challenge. First mentioned by Chris Bloor in his book, *The Inner Path – Closer to the Countryside*, the intention of the Green Man Challenge was to introduce more people to the countryside around Bristol by completing an entire circuit of the Community Forest Path between dawn and dusk. The challenge can be undertaken at any time of the year, alone or in a group and isn't run as an organised event. The Green Man Ultra, organised by Steve Worrallo at Ultra Running, took this same basic challenge but ran the whole thing under race conditions, with an official 15 hour cut-off. You paid your entry fee, you got a number and if you finished in time then you got a medal and a t-shirt. But it wasn't only material possessions that could be gleaned from completing the event – finishing the course in under twenty-four hours automatically gave you the right to become a Woodwose and have your name entered in the *Forestal Book of the Honourable Order of Woodwoses*.

Not being forest-wise, I didn't honestly know what a Woodwose was, so I wasn't really sure whether to be impressed by that or not. It could be that having an extra Mars bar in the goody bag would be a more useful option after running forty-six miles. After a bit of reading up on all things mythical and forest-like, I discovered that a Woodwose was apparently a savage form of hairy humanoid that links mortals with the dangerous spirits of the woodland – a bit like a crazed David Bellamy.

Originally seen as a wild and darksome protector of the forests of medieval Europe, in today's secular and cynical times he would more likely be viewed as a feral anti-road campaigner who'd been holed up in a tree for a decade without realising the bypass had already opened. In fact some people originally believed the Woodwose to be merely humans who escaped to the woodland, turning wild and growing their hair long for survival, while others thought they could have even been remnants of Neanderthals living in Europe at the time. In North America the same basic legends were manifested by the tale of Bigfoot, who depending upon your age and viewing choice either a) got hit by a car and went to live with the Hendersons, or b) was defeated by the Six Million Dollar Man in *The Secret of Bigfoot* (although that Bigfoot turned out to be a robot created by aliens living inside a Californian mountain, for reasons never fully explained). Either way, he was not quite the wild protector of the forest as he was back in Europe.

Thinking about it all for a little while I wasn't so sure that my thinning hair would grow long enough anymore to do the whole Woodwose thing justice, and even if it did it would all be white. I'd be a winter Woodwose. It would obviously be nice to gain a formal title but I'm not sure that it would go well on a business card. According to the event website you could also earn the right to be named as a Wistman if you set a course record, or if your achievement suggested you had some of the magical qualities associated with the term. Quite what magical qualities they were after it didn't say, but I knew I was crap at card tricks (I can't even shuffle properly) and there was no way I was going to be breaking any course records unless I got a bus between checkpoints, so I wasn't too worried about earning this.

No, without wanting to sound really ungrateful or disrespectful to the ancient spiritual ways of the forest or the history of the path, but if I'd just run all the way around Greater Bristol between dawn and dusk, then I'm not really going to be too bothered earning the right to be called something that made me sound like an extra from Lord of the Rings. What I would want more than anything would be a plain white t-shirt with massive bold red print on it saying: *"I just ran 46 f**king miles!"* Granted it's not a common design for race t-shirts but I'm sure it would be a good talking point.

So with the knowledge of the what and where of the Green Man in the bank, I needed to start working out exactly how I was going to tackle such a huge challenge. How did I go about training for an ultramarathon? How could I learn and remember the entire route? How could I persuade the organisers of my t-shirt design? I decided the starting point for all these questions was to make a call to the only actual real-life Woodwose I knew – listed in the *Forestal Book of H.O.O.W.* as number fifty-six, Bill Graham.

3. With a Little Help from My Friends

"The only source of knowledge is experience." – **Albert Einstein**

It was Saturday April 22nd 2006 and I was standing in a bar in Hammersmith, West London thinking I should probably be in bed already. It was all of about nine o'clock, but on the night before I was due to run my first marathon I stood there nervously sipping a diet coke wondering how Bill Graham was jovially enjoying a pint of Guinness without a care in the world. My head was filled with a million and one things I had read about how best to prepare for a marathon and dancing around drinking beer certainly wasn't on any list or in any magazine article I had seen. The conformist side of my brain was worried for him, hoping it really didn't all come back to bite him the next day, but he seemed totally oblivious to his reckless pre-race behaviour. The following morning we all got up, had breakfast in the hotel, took the coach to Blackheath and ran the 26th Flora London Marathon. Bill, aged 52, ran home in a spritely 2 hours 50 minutes, taking 16th in his age category and 575th place overall. I on the other hand stumbled around in a painful 4 hours 6 minutes, finishing in 13,156th. As we sat on the coach back to Bristol that evening, my legs totally destroyed, I decided never to question Bill's approach to running again.

I first met Bill Graham when I joined Bitton Road Runners, back in 2005, and had got to know him pretty well through his many roles at the club. Over the years as a member he had transitioned seamlessly from regular club runner, through England Athletics trained coach, men's captain, to head coach and even a stepping up under difficult circumstances to put in a stint as club chairman. I always had a lot of time for Bill as he always had plenty of time and patience for others and was often the calm voice of experience and reason. It was Bill, through his coaching and advice that had helped me achieve some of my best times in races over the years and right now he seemed like the best person to speak to about surviving my first ultramarathon. Particularly given it was one he had already run, coming in fourth the previous year, taking the veteran prize with his time of 8 hours straight.

Already an experienced distance runner in his fifties by the time I met him, Bill had spent several years successfully running cross country at school and county level during the late 1960s before emigrating to South Africa, where due to the fact his school wasn't big on sport, he switched to playing football and running went on hold. By 1982, living back in the UK and suffering from knee problems, it was suggested he start running between matches to see if it helped. Not only did it help but it also reignited his passion for running and he quickly became enticed by the challenge of testing himself over the 26.2 miles of a marathon. He completed his first in Winchester in 1982 with a respectable performance of 3 hours 45 minutes and was instantly hooked. Years of hard training combined with lots of trial and error saw him smash his marathon best down to 2 hours 35 minutes in 1990 and his half marathon time down to just 71 minutes the following year. During the late 1990s, realising his peak speeds were behind him he stepped up his mileage and started to take on bigger and more varied challenges. Having already run the popular fifty-six mile Comrades Marathon in South Africa (think double length London Marathon in the sun) during the 1980s, ultra distance running wasn't a complete unknown and he soon switched to running mountain marathons and ultras.

Whilst age might have robbed him of some of his youthful speed, he found it had given in return a greater patience to control his pace, enabling him to cover distances much further than before. He moved away from road racing and took on events such as The Josh Naylor Challenge (forty-eight miles and 17,000 feet of ascent in the Lake District), The High Peak Marathon (forty miles around the Peak District) and obviously, The Green Man Ultra. If anybody was in a position to help me get through this challenge, it was Bill.

With the race entry in, steely determination set and the clock ticking, I made a call to Bill and arranged to pop around to his house and discuss the race, the route and generally how to go about running forty-six miles and surviving. It was September 13th, the day after my (and coincidentally Bill's) birthday when I rolled up outside his front door hungry for knowledge. Alongside me my running partner, associate challenge sucker and fellow budding Green Man novice: Bear Schlenker.

I should state at this point that whilst quite a friendly and cuddly moniker, Bear was not actually his real name, but was one that had been given to him (mostly by me) because of his numerous woodland activities whilst out running – not those of the adventurer type, more of the call of nature type. If I'm honest, it was a juvenile nickname at best but unfortunately for him it was one that had stuck. Now, when he was looking after somebody he became Care Bear; when he was grumpy he was Grizzly Bear; and when he was cold he simply became Polar Bear. It was the name that just kept on giving. For the record, Bear's real name was in fact Rudi, although in certain circles that has long been discarded in favour of Bear. So much so that even his girlfriend now called him Bear. To be fair to Bear, it was he who christened me Bumblebee in the first place, so I think we were actually kind of quits.

The Green Man was to be Bear's first ultramarathon too, and regardless of the fact that he'd naturally be more at home in the woods, he was just as anxious as I was with how we were going to tackle it. Unlike my many years running, Bear had only been pounding his paws on the streets for little more than eighteen months by the time we talked each other into becoming ultramarathon runners. Despite his relatively short time running he had already ramped his racing mileage up from the Bristol 10K to the Paris Marathon in less than a year (although a particularly nasty salad poisoning incident meant he left more than his enduring legacy on the streets of the French capital), proving if nothing else his dedication to training and a sense of stoic determination, both important attributes for taking on ultra distances. More importantly, Bear was a methodical realist which would help temper my overly confident mindset throughout our training and race preparation. A touch of sanity to help keep my delusions rooted close to ground level.

Crowding round one end of Bill's large wooden dining table that September evening the three of us stared fixedly at the laptop screen as he clicked, dragged and narrated his way through what seemed like an endless amount of aerial photography, detailing the worryingly long and largely rural route. Online mapping is such an incredible resource and had quickly become my default way to plan out training runs. Whereas in the good old days I would just guess the distance based upon how long I was out running or by measuring it first by driving it in a car, nowadays thanks to the power of websites like Mapometer* you can work out exactly how far your run is, where you have to turn and what landmarks to look for along the way all without even leaving the sofa. The downside to all this power of being able to snoop into people's back gardens to see what patio furniture they had two years ago is that it can overwhelm you with information if you're not careful. Moving around the

---

* http://www.mapometer.com – by far the simplest and best online mapping tool in my opinion.

Community Forest Path mile by mile, Bill handed down his learned wisdom of each and every section with such speed and depth of knowledge you couldn't help but be impressed. From the start of the race at the Redwood Hotel we whizzed down to the Ashton Court Estate and out the other side, under the A370, through woods, ditches and fields up to the A38, diving behind the hotel, and up over the fields climbing to the very top of the Dundry hills. Speeding past the radio transmitters we tumbled down through numerous farms and villages I'd never heard of, still following the path, all the way across fields and bridges, over hills and stiles, until we finally hit the Norton Malreward village hall – all that and you're still only just shy of ten miles in at checkpoint one. Every time Bill zoomed in on a particular point and gave us specifics of which part of the hedge to look for the kissing gate in, or which side of which trees to pass through, or even which of the path's direction signs to actually ignore, I nodded with an affirmative *"uh-ha"* and made a mental note, recording each miniscule fact for precise recall when out on the route. The biggest problem with this however was that my mental note-taking capacity is incredibly low and within a few short minutes I was already recycling the notepad and overwriting pages I had used at the start. Every now and then I would look around at Bear and see a distant look in his glazed eyes – I think we lost him in a ditch somewhere around the A38. As somebody who often walks into a room and forgets what they went in there for in the first place, I wondered exactly how I was going to remember forty-six miles of kissing gates, fields and hidden gaps between trees. There was no doubt that Bill's intimate knowledge of the course was going to be helpful, but trying to learn and remember it all in one evening was clearly a fruitless task.

As luck would have it, being just one day after my birthday, I had been given quite possibly the most nerdish present ever – a pair of Ordnance Survey maps covering the entire route. Never before had I been so genuinely excited to receive a map as a gift and hopefully never will again. Opening them out all over the dining table I was even more excited to see that the Community Forest Path was actually already marked out. It made it look all official and somehow more real. I took out a child-size pink highlighter pen and illuminated the path to make it stand out more clearly for tired eyes. Once I'd coloured in the entire loop we all stood back and looked over the huge unfolded map and took in the sheer scale of it all. Being born and having grown up in Bristol many of the place names the highlighter line passed through were familiar to me and I could visualise the areas, but seeing just how many of these places I would be passing through over the course of a single run, was daunting. Up until this point it had all been talk but here it was laid out in bright pink in front of us in all its 1:25000 scale reality. I laughed nervously wondering how the hell I was going to be able to run that far. Having run a few marathons I knew what it was like to suffer over long distances and knew how I felt after twenty-six miles, how was I going to keep it going for another twenty on top of that? At that point the whole thing just seemed slightly stupid and quite impossible. But that was when I was looking at it from the perspective of a road runner.

After Bill had finished his flyover of the path, we sat and talked trails, tips and tactics, and it all started to make a little bit more sense. When you're running in a road race it's all about the time. You're running against the clock and you push yourself hard to achieve a goal of a certain time. It's not about winning, it's about knocking minutes, even sometimes mere seconds off your previous best. It's not even right really to call it a race, as a race is something that you actually stand a chance of winning. You can consider yourself as having been in a race if you break the tape by pushing out of your chest as you fall over the line to a hero's applause, safe in the knowledge that there was nobody else in front of you when you finally stopped. You were first and the next guy was second. That is a race. Out of all the events I've ever entered, I can count the number of actual races I've been in on one hand, using a thumb. I remember it well. It was July 2009, my daughter's reception class sports day – the dad's race. Approximately one-hundred metres of sheer testosterone-fuelled bravado played out in front of a horde of proud children and disparaging wives. Jokes and banter filled the air as the over-willing volunteers made their way to the start, all playing down their own sprinting prowess whilst simultaneously stretching and checking their laces. As luck would have it I appeared to somehow be wearing my running shoes that day, not that I was alone. Once in place the jollity died down and the starting line-up, which resembled less an athletic grouping and more a queue for the chip shop, fell silent. I took a quick look up and down the line, sizing up my opponents, seeing who was going to be finishing behind me. I was pretty confident. I saw myself as something of a wolf in sheep's clothing – a sprinter extraordinaire hidden in plain sight, my raw talent masked by my large frame and sizeable stomach. My self-confidence stemmed from my recent bouts of track speedwork, which had been going pretty well, so long as we didn't run over four-hundred metres, as that was the point where my powerful legs lost the battle to power my very unsprinter-like physique. My only obvious contender in the event was a fellow dad who I knew to be a triathlete, and who was also considerably slimmer and fitter looking than me. I however had the element of surprise on my side. Nobody expected to be beaten in a sprint by a fat man even if he was wearing a Paris Half Marathon t-shirt (in extra-large). On your marks, get set, GO bellowed the headmaster and we powered off the line to a cacophony of excited shouting and cheering from the gathered supporters. My wife however stood with her slowly shaking head in her hands. She of all people knew my mindset. She knew that I am one of the least competitive people alive – unless I actually think I have a chance of winning, when I will go all out guns blazing – and that day I had the faith. The race itself was something of a blur and short of my legs starting to give out under me at around eighty metres I was unaware of anything happening around me. I had tunnel vision for the finish line, which could have been either sheer focus or a lack of blood to my optic nerves. As we hit the line in a time Jamaican sprinters would only use as an insult, my vision restored and I became aware there was nobody in front of me. I was first, by a belly. It was close, but victory was mine, much to the amazement of spectators and fellow runners alike. There were no medals that day, and no congratulations from triathlete dad but I didn't need any of that, I was a winner. My kids thought I was amazing, my wife thought I was mental and I just thought I'm glad that it was over. I haven't won a race since then, I'm just not that good a runner and I'm OK with that. I've got a shoebox full of finisher medals in the loft and even got a few certificates tucked away somewhere but I certainly didn't win any of them, I was merely handed them for finishing, like a memento of the day.

Unless you are an extreme athlete of the very highest calibre then running an ultramarathon is certainly never going to be a race and nor is it even going to really be about the time. OK, being honest, it will always be a little bit about the time, in so much as you will probably set out with a target in mind but the reality is that it's not the type of event where your pace or splits* have any real significance. One of the first nuggets of information Bill handed over during our post-route briefing was the fact that we shouldn't even consider running the entire thing. The best thing to do was set out with a strategy and a common one was to walk anything that looked like a hill. That came as something of a surprise; because when you're pounding the streets in a road race the idea of planning

---

* Total running time broken down into time chunks relevant to your run, such as per mile or per lap.

to incorporate a few strolls into your run would be personal best (PB) suicide. Unless you were shattered walking was always a big no-no but here we were being told to plan to walk from the start. The concept though was simple; the idea of factoring in walking uphill is quite simply to conserve energy, because you're going to need buckets of it to keep going over the extreme distance. Any small time advantage you could possibly gain from running up the hills would be paid for by the excessive energy you would waste by doing it. Sure, if you were an elite athlete you wouldn't consider doing anything but running every inch of the course, but for most people who undertake ultras, walking is always going to be part of the deal. As much as the road runner in me thought it sounded defeatist, I could see the logic in it.

What became clear after talking with Bill for a couple of hours was that running an ultramarathon was a lot more about endurance and getting to the finish than it was about the actual time you finished in. It was more about survival than speed. The overall pace of running such an event is much slower than you would run in a road race, but given the distances and often difficult terrain involved, there's no way you could possibly compare the two. And there is the crux of it – what we learnt that evening was to forget everything we thought we knew about running a race that we'd learnt from the road or track, because this was a different beast entirely. Forget the head down watching your pace; forget the even splits; forget the mile markers, the pacers, forget it all. This was solely about endurance; keeping energy levels up by eating as you're going; conserving energy by walking the steep bits; and most of all just keep putting one foot in front of the other, at any speed, until you finished. By the time we were ready to leave both Bear and myself had gone through the full gamut of emotions from trepidation, through fear, ending up on wistful. We'd seen the route, we'd been briefed with insider knowledge and we'd got to do some colouring in on a map. We were ready to start our training.

4. Putting Yourself to the Test

"Whether you think you can, or think you can't, you're right."
– **Henry Ford**

September was coming to a close and following our meeting with Bill a couple of weeks earlier I had started to formulate a rough training plan. It had to be fairly loose as I could never rigidly follow a schedule, mostly because running always had to fit in around everything else that was going on. A careful balancing of family life, work and training – which being honest I didn't always get right. It's a familiar juggling act for many runners, particularly when training for anything of any significant distance, so quite how I would find the time to build up my endurance to run forty-six miles I wasn't quite sure. I didn't even really know how far I should run in training. Bill's sage advice was that time on your feet was the most important thing. Forget miles and just get used to being on your feet for long periods of time, keeping going when you're tired and really want to quit. In terms of distance, just as in the build up to a marathon you don't actually run twenty-six miles, you're never going to run the whole distance of an ultra in training, covering up to about thirty miles would be enough in this case.

The peak of the training schedule was to be a back-to-back weekender. This is where we would split the race distance into two relatively even chunks and run one half on Saturday and the other on Sunday. It sounded pretty brutal, running almost a marathon on Saturday and then the same again the very next day – it was the kind of thing you read about in books. But hey, that was months away so we could forget about it for now, like it wasn't actually ever going to happen. Bill assured us that if we could pull that off then we would be fine on the day. I liked his optimism but at the end of September when I was still pretty fat and rather unfit it all still seemed very hypothetical – both the distances and the time we would need to spend out running. Our pluck-a-time-out-of-the-air target for the ultra had been set at completing it less than 10 hours. Why less than 10? Well, simply because 9 hours something is still in single figures, nothing more complicated or scientific than that. Not because that's the time we could carry enough food for, or because that's when it would be getting dark, or even because my shoes would turn back into pumpkins when the clock struck 10 hours. No, just because it was still in single digits and looked better on paper. It was a loose goal which was helpful to have to work towards rather than just going out with no idea. At that point however I didn't think I could even stand up for 10 hours straight, let alone keep moving for that long. There was certainly a lot of work to be done.

Taking Bill's advice on board my plan was quite straightforward and that was basically to try and run lots of miles. Run through the week, lunchtimes or running into work (sometimes both), some hill training for strength, some off-road running to get used to the terrain and steadily increasing the distance of the long weekend run. Along the way we would also learn the Green Man route as much as possible by breaking it down into manageable chunks and running them by following the nice pink line on the map – reconnaissance missions to help us better get to grips with our muddy foe. The last thing we needed to be worrying about on race day was which way was the right way. We needed to know the route intimately, making navigation second nature.

Alongside all the miles I would cut right back on the booze and stop eating the cakes, sweets and junk that had come to be normality between meals. Largely the meals I ate at home were fairly healthy; it was mostly I just ate too much of them, as well as too much other rubbish, like takeaways for breakfast; slipping in an extra sandwich or perhaps a pasty at lunchtime; chocolate bars and cakes in the afternoon. It all had to stop. I adopted the mindset that I wasn't going on any kind of fad diet or depriving myself of anything, I was just going to have a bit less of everything and make sensible choices. After many years of attempting to lose weight I understood the basics of my calorific needs, the calorie and fat content of most foods and drinks I consumed and the kind of energy I would expend from running lots of miles. As simple as it sounds all you really need to do to lose weight is eat healthily and exercise plenty. It is after all basic science – you need to use more energy than you put back in (alright, there is a touch more to it than that, Google it if you want to find out the finer details).

With five months until the race I wondered if science could help me with my challenge even more. Just as in the opening titles of *The Six Million Dollar Man* where Steve Austin is put through his paces on a treadmill with scientists tweaking his bionic programming, could I somehow be analysed and tweaked to run better – even without my childhood bionics? Better is a very subjective term, I guess what I was after was something that would help make my training more specific, more focused on ultra distances. It would also be interesting to measure how fit, or rather unfit, I was before and then again after the training. Hopefully seeing a big change in fitness on paper as well as in my running would surely help with the psychological side of the challenge. Despite my chunky frame at the time, I had been doing bits of running through the summer, although nothing with any real speed, structure or purpose; it was all very much the flight of the bumblebee.

Investigating the subject of sport science more, I came across the website of the University of Bath and the rather grandiose sounding Human Performance Centre. That sounded ideal. Open to professional sportsmen and women, the general public and bumblebees alike, I dropped them an email to find out more about how they could help me in my quest. A couple of days later I received a very positive reply from the chief sport scientist at the centre, Jonathan Robinson, outlining how he thought they would be able to help me. The first test he suggested was a body composition test. This essentially determines how much of your body is actually made up of fat. Not whether or not you were fat, as everyone should have some element of fat to them, it's how much of you actually is fat that is the important bit. I liked the sound of the test but wasn't sure if I would be so keen to hear the results. I wondered if their equipment went up to OMG. The next tests Jonathan recommended were VO_2 max and lactate threshold. These look at your fitness by measuring the amount of oxygen you use when running and how lactate builds up in your blood during a run. Using the results from these they would be able to compile a heart rate based training guide, specifically tailored for me, which would help target my training at a specific event, in this case the ultra and my endurance generally. Both of these tests would be carried out as I ran at a steadily increasing pace on a treadmill while a machine analysed my breathing and somebody took blood samples, measuring the lactate build-up. It all sounded very scientific and exactly what I was after, so I took the next available slot, which was a couple of weeks away. In the meantime I would carry on with the start of my training as originally planned and the plan for that weekend was to run the Bristol Half Marathon.

Running a half marathon at this point was going to be a test in itself, as I was in no real shape to be doing it let alone getting a time I would ever be happy with. But that was if I was running the race for myself, which this time around I wasn't. Having run the Bristol Half Marathon about six or seven times in the past I was

and wouldn't go back on that promise. I wasn't particularly looking forward to it yet nor was I worried about it. My ever-confident brain told me I could run thirteen miles no problem, I'd done it loads of times; the question was just how long that run would take. Having only recently started my new regime of training and eating it was still very early days and weighing in at 16st 6lb, I was, as far as I could remember, the heaviest I had ever been when running a race. Also, for the first time in seven years of running with Bitton Road Runners, I stood on the start line of a race not wearing my blue and yellow club vest. If I'm honest, that was partly due to the fact that because I knew I wouldn't run a time I would be happy with, I would rather do it quietly and secondly - and probably more importantly - it just didn't fit. Sure I could get it on, but despite being an extra-large it was still a pretty tight fit. I felt uncomfortable wearing it. Not in an overtly snug way but because I knew I was fat and it did nothing but highlight that simple fact. Lately I had found myself wearing increasingly baggier clothes to hide in, rather than those that were more fitted (and bulging). Trying to stay anonymous in Bristol however was a fruitless task as I was quickly spotted by many fellow club members, all of whom enquired as to why I wasn't wearing my vest. One runner even spotted me in the starting crowd identifying me from the back of my head. I didn't ask him how.

The race went off pretty much to plan and I kept Tim on track by pacing him to run each mile steadily at nine minutes which, as long as we stuck to that, would get us in just under the magical 2 hour mark. Keeping the pace down at the start of the race, while everyone else rushed off too fast, we stayed steady settling into a rhythm out along the long straight Portway and then back down the other side. We were ticking the miles off seemingly with ease and despite his lack of experience Tim was a strong runner with solid determination and was keeping the pace up without any real trouble. It was as we were coming up to Castle Park at about the eleven mile mark that I found myself starting to flag and a thought flashed through my head of Tim getting in under two hours on his own and me struggling to finish. I kept it to myself, gritted my teeth and ran on, over Bristol Bridge, looping back by St. Mary Redcliffe, through Queen Square and out onto the City Centre coming up on the final mile marker. Running around the centre and heading down towards the back of the Watershed is such a great feeling when you know you are on course for your target time. At that point I told Tim to kick it up a gear and we would smash the two hour mark in the face. Sprinting, we weaved in and out of people to the finish line on Anchor Road, crossing the timing mat in a time of 1 hour 57 minutes. It was a great result. I was pleased for Tim having achieved his goal, despite the fact that I now owed him lunch, but I was also secretly pleased for myself for managing to get around in under two hours, something I wasn't that confident of at the start of the day. The surprising thing is that while I might have been the heaviest I had ever been running a race, amazingly I had run worse times in the past. The bumblebee was clearly in better shape than I realised. Exactly what kind of shape, I would soon find out.

Two weeks later, on a dull Tuesday afternoon, I parked in the car park on campus at the University of Bath and walked through the impressive sports complex to meet the director of the Human Performance Centre, Jonathan Robinson. We talked about my ultramarathon challenge as we walked and he took me through a set of corridors to a small nondescript room overlooking the Olympic-sized swimming pool that could almost have doubled as a spare storeroom. It wasn't very big, nor was it filled with lots of computers, flashing lights, or boffins in white coats. But this apparently was where all the magic happened, where science made good men great, where sport superstars were born. Somehow, I kind of expected more, although maybe I'd just been watching too many films. Almost filling the small room was an assorted collection of exercise equipment making it look like a slightly crap gym. At the back and dominating the room was an industrial size treadmill which had a large arch reaching over the top of it with a rope attached. This was apparently to attach a safety harness to when people were running. Why would you need that? Well the treadmill will hit speeds up to 40kph that's why. A touch faster than anything at any gym I've ever been to. In fact I've had cars that would have struggled to keep up with that. Jonathan told me about how in the run-up to the 2012 London Olympics they had had the Saint Vincent and The Grenadines sprinters in there knocking out reps at around 35kph – scary. The rest of the room was filled by a rowing machine and a couple of exercise bikes of sorts. Around the edges of the room on benches there were a handful of computers at which people were working. As well as Jonathan and myself, there were three students (two Abby's and a Luke) in the room who were all on work placements for their degree courses, and would be helping with my testing.

So here I was ready to be tested. What had seemed like a good idea a month or so ago however I wasn't now quite so sure of. These people were scientists, professionals who worked with professional sportsmen and women. As was my way I hadn't really put much thought to it until now, until I turned up and walked into the room, but now I was wondering if I actually deserved to be there. I wasn't an athlete, I was just a bumblebee. Were they secretly sniggering behind my back at the fat guy who wanted to be tested, playing at being an athlete? Did I even need to be here? Didn't I just need to put down the pies and beer and get out there putting one foot in front of another? Ultimately I'm a great believer in asking for help when you need it. It's not possible to know everything in life, so accepting that means you need to know when to ask somebody else how to best do something. Just like I'd already asked Bill for his help, I was now using the fact that money can buy you many things in life and here I was buying some professional sporting scientific help. Deserve didn't come into it. If somebody has the desire to learn and the funds by which to settle the bill, then the expertise the centre offers is as applicable and relevant to them as it would be to the highest of sports stars. Obviously I could just get out there and train hard for five months, or I could spend a few quid, use science and Jonathan's fifteen years of experience to help make my training smarter and more focussed. The two were very different.

I took off the vest and tracksuit trousers I had been hiding in and we started off with the basics, height and weight. As expected, I was still six feet tall and jumping on their scales, I weighed in at a chunky 15st 12lb. Clearly my cut-back programme had been working fairly well over the first few weeks with a loss of 8lb so far. I was pretty happy with that. Next we moved onto the body composition test. This involved Jonathan making measurements in seven places down the right-hand side of my body and drawing crosses with a marker pen at the centre point of key areas such as my forearm, thigh and dreaded belly. Then using a pair of skinfold callipers (or fat grapplers as I like to call them) he pinched the flab on the crosses and wrote down a bunch of numbers. I didn't see exactly what he was writing down but I could've sworn though at one point I saw him gently shaking his head whilst sucking air in through his teeth. From the measurements taken and the calliper readings he would be able to work out what percentage of my body was made up of fat.

Sticking my vest back on I jumped onto the treadmill and jogged for five minutes to warm up before the other tests began. I was wearing a heart rate belt around my chest that was linked to a monitor, telling the testing team how fast my heart was pumping. Once warmed up, I donned a face mask covering my nose and mouth with a tight seal and had a small blood sample taken to measure my baseline lactate level. The test was explained as a continual run with speed increasing by 1kph every three minutes.

During each repetition my breathing would be analysed for the amount of oxygen and carbon dioxide I inhaled and exhaled. At the end of each rep, before the speed increased, my blood would be taken and tested and the lactate level recorded. The idea was to keep running for as long as possible, recording the measurements at the end of each three minute rep. Your VO_2 max is reached when the amount of oxygen being used remains the same despite increasing effort. This is the maximum capacity of your body to transport and use oxygen during exercise and is commonly used to indicate your level of fitness. The blood taken would be tested to monitor the lactate build up and determine my lactate threshold. Without getting too scientific, lactate is a by-product of your body burning energy during exercise. As it builds up in your blood it is generally recycled by your body, keeping the levels under control – but only up to a certain point. That point is your threshold. Past this point levels of lactate in your blood rise more significantly as it cannot be reused (commonly known to runners as lactic acid build-up). This causes muscle fatigue and ultimately exhaustion.

Starting off the first few efforts were pretty light jogs, with the treadmill starting at 8kph. After each rep I would also be asked to indicate on a chart my RPE (rate of perceived exertion), which would be recorded along with the other data. The first few were quite casual and easy going and my RPE score reflected that. On the fifth rep with the treadmill running at 12kph (about eight minutes per mile) the jocularity had gone and we were into proper running territory. I had now been running for around fifteen minutes and with each rep my RPE was noticeably increasing alongside the speed. I could see if I glanced over at the computer screen my oxygen usage starting to rise steeply too. Every kph speed increase now would mean a jump of around thirty seconds per mile at a time when I was starting to flag and the running was getting tougher. I ran through the sixth rep at 13kph with my eyes firmly on the next one, and when we got to the seventh as the treadmill lurched up to 14kph, I pounded the belt determined to finish not just this rep but the next one too. In hindsight it's easy to see why I was really starting to suffer at this point as I had been running for over twenty minutes and was now running a sub seven minute mile pace. No wonder it was starting to hurt. The treadmill sped up again to 15kph and after the blood had been taken I jumped back on the moving belt with a solid determination to make it to 16kph. I ran, with sweat rolling down my face and back, trying to focus on anything in the small room that would distract my mind from what I was asking my body to do. I kept pushing and pushing thinking the end must be close, ready to stop at any second, when I heard Jonathan shout what I'm sure he meant as an encouraging message of *"Well done, only just over a minute left to go"* – a minute? I thought I was there. His message of goodwill almost broke me; I dug deep and kept my legs moving through the final agonising seconds until the rep was complete. I stood on the side of the treadmill with my legs barely able to hold me up as Abby took more blood from my finger and thought whether or not I could complete another rep at 16kph. With salty sweat running into and stinging my eyes I decided not and hit the stop button. Nearly twenty-eight minutes in and I was done. I sat down on a stool, a fat sweaty panting wreck. I had also made the mistake of giving my phone to Jonathan to take some pictures of me during the test on the camera and looking back at them later he seems to have captured well a balding, sweaty, fat man trying to run fast on a treadmill. It wasn't a pretty sight, but in the immortal words of Bucks Fizz: *"My camera never lies"*. They would serve their purpose well as the before shot, from a before and after montage. Now all I had to do was wait for Jonathan to analyse all the results, compile my report and send it over.

5. Getting Results

"Superhuman effort isn't worth a damn unless it achieves results."
– Ernest Shackleton

On the Discovery channel there's a show called *Stan Lee's Superhumans* in which they travel the planet in search of individuals who have incredible and unusual abilities. Stan Lee should know all about such things, given he was the co-creator of some of the biggest superhero names in the Marvel Universe such as the X-Men, Spiderman and Iron Man to name but a few. The idea behind the programme is to show that through evolution and mutation it is possible for real people to have, what could be seen as, superhuman abilities. In one episode I saw they covered Ultramarathon Man himself, Dean Karnazes. The show started by following Karnazes on a leisurely twelve hour run where he covered eighty miles (that's running a nine minute mile average), before stopping for a brief chat and then running a further thirty miles back home to San Francisco. Later in the show they took him to a sport science lab and put him on a treadmill to test his blood lactate, in the same way that I had been tested in Bath. What they found, to the astonishment of the sport scientists was that as Karnazes kept running his blood lactate did not rise, hovering for the most part around 2.1 mmol, in fact at one point later in the run it actually started to fall. What this meant was that his body was able to deal with the lactic acid as it was being produced and because it wasn't building up his muscles didn't fatigue or cramp anywhere near the same amount as those of a mere mortal undertaking the same task. Whether or not this was some form of a genetic mutation remains to be seen but it did explain some of how Karnazes could run such long distances, seemingly with ease.

Within a week of undergoing my tests in Bath, as promised, an email rolled into my inbox with my performance report and training guidance attached. As I downloaded and opened the Word document I wondered if my lactate levels would match Karnazes, or perhaps I might even be better. Skimming through the twelve pages of graphs, charts and numbers I didn't spot the words *'amazing'*; *'superhuman'*; or even *'incredible'* anywhere. On a second skimming I did spot *'not too bad considering'*; *'reasonably well developed'*; and *'good levels of strength and determination'*, which for a fat man in his forties I took as being pretty good going. As well as the blood lactate figures what I was interested in was technically how fat I was, the VO_2 max result and how I could best target my training for the ultra.

I had started my weight loss and training plan with the Bristol Half Marathon the month before at a sturdy weight of 16st 6lbs, which gave me a Body Mass Index (BMI) of 31.2 – firmly within the obese range. The problem with BMI though is that it is just a simple height by weight calculation*, not taking into account things like amount of muscle or waist size. Somebody could train for months, lose fat and gain muscle but remain the same weight and still be in an unfavourable BMI bracket. The BMI system of measurement was devised in 1832 as a simple means to determine the thickness or thinness of people. It was never designed to indicate how much fat somebody has, despite that being how it is commonly interpreted today. This is why I decided to undergo a body composition test at the Human Performance Centre, to get a proper diagnosis. The average body fat percentage for a man depends entirely on who you ask but using World Health Organisation (WHO) recommendations, a

* bmi = mass(kg)/(height(m))2

healthy man in his forties should be somewhere in the range of 11-22%, with athletic types generally having lower body fat, normally around the 7-15% mark. Reading through my report from Jonathan I came across the body composition section and there, below a table of measurements was my percentage: 21.1%. Wow. I had to check it again to make sure that it wasn't being halved or something, but no it was correct. How could I be so fat and yet actually not be fat at all in the eyes of the WHO? According to my BMI I was obese and yet the WHO were telling me I was (just) within the normal range for a man of my age. It could have been a bit lower if I was more athletic but I wasn't – I was a bumblebee. What the breakdown of body measurements in the report highlighted was that whilst my entire body fat was in the normal range, my abdominal region was chocked full of blubber – a classic beer belly – and was where my problem obviously lay. Overall it wasn't quite what I was expecting, but through a positive interpretation of the numbers it was a small psychological boost. Forget the fat magnet waist-band and go by the numbers alone and I was almost normal.

I moved onto the treadmill test covering the VO_2 max and blood lactate. The first graph I came across showed my lactate measuring 1.8 mmol at the start of the test, before dropping slightly to 1.6, then rising again through 2.2; 2.9; 3.9; 5.6; and finally ending the test on 7.8 – each measurement being between the speed rep increases on the treadmill when my blood was taken. Clearly I was no Karnazes, where his lactate balanced out at 2.1 throughout, mine rocketed up after the going started to get tough. With a treadmill speed of 15kph and a heart rate of 187bpm I wasn't surprised to see the steep climb towards the end of the test – I was a wreck by the time we finished and could barely stand.

Whilst I was a broken man at the end of the test, again all was not lost. In the report Jonathan had written: "*You currently display quite a good aerobic profile considering your background which is*

twist it too far though; it was a pretty good outcome. A relative VO$_2$ max score of 48.0 ml/kg/min is actually pretty good, putting me well above average and close to excellent for my age. Even better was that relative scores are recorded as millilitres per kilogram per minute, which means that it is possible to improve your VO$_2$ max simply by losing weight, which was obviously all part of my grand plan.

Sitting back in my chair with the report open on the screen it dawned on me that I wasn't actually in as bad shape as I thought I was. Sure I was fat around the middle and a world away from being an elite runner, but I was expecting much worse results. The report showed that my blood lactate wasn't particularly high at the end of the test, which highlighted (in Jonathan's words) *"significant aerobic development that clearly exists in your physiology"*. All the years running as the bumblebee had had a positive effect, even on my fat lazy body. As well as promising lactate levels and an above average VO$_2$ max score, the tests also highlighted that I had good running economy. Running economy is measured by how much oxygen your body uses when running. This becomes more vital as the distance over which you run increases, so clearly the lower score here the better. My average running economy across all the speeds tested was 205.93 ml/kg/km, which was apparently of quite a good level considering what I was aiming to achieve and my recent background. Elite endurance runners would usually elicit scores of below 200 ml/kg/km, so it wasn't too shabby a score here either.

This all moved the goalposts slightly. I went into the test thinking the report was going to out me as some kind of pie-eating sloth who had no chance at all of pulling the whole thing off. The reality however was something different and because of that my perspective of the whole challenge had changed. Instead of being a fat runner who was going to try desperately to tackle an ultramarathon, fighting to get around and survive, now I was a semi-fat runner who through the use of science had discovered that he was fitter and more capable than he thought and with a bit of effort and hard work could probably make a reasonable distance runner. It's funny, because I'd always considered myself better as a shorter distance runner, as although I was carrying a bulk my powerful legs would allow me to sprint quickly over short distances when pushed. This report however blew that apart and made me realise that with some specific training and obviously weight loss from my lard belt, I could actually be quite good at this. I guess it's all about perception and belief. At that point the delusional part of my brain took over and pictured me running hundred mile races with ease. I was planning how I would get into the Western States 100 even before I had really started training for the Green Man, let alone run it.

The report had served its purpose well, not only had it set down a baseline for me to measure my training against but it had highlighted the fact that I was more suited and capable at running long distances than I ever realised, and having scientific proof of that was a strong weapon when it came to the mental battle of distance running. It also laid out heart rate training zones that I should train within to flatten out that lactate graph and get my body geared up for a bloody long run. It was pretty simple stuff, train wearing a heart rate monitor and try to keep my heart within a certain range for most of the training and that would help build my endurance. All in, it was a great report and fired me up ready for training to really begin.

6. Training Diary: October

"The way to get started is to quit talking and begin doing"
– Walt Disney

Total Miles Run: 156.75
Highest Weekly Total: 44.75
Weekly Average: 35.39

Starting training in October was exciting. After all the thinking, talking and planning here we were finally getting out there and treading ground in preparation for the big day just five months away. For the most part my training runs would consist of lunchtime jaunts from the office in and around Bath, as well as runs both into, and home from work, all backed up by a long weekend run to build endurance. I had treated myself to a new pair of Mizuno Wave Inspire which were my road shoes of choice, as well as a pair of Adidas Kanadia for the off-road days. The Adidas were a hybrid trail shoe rather than a full-on off-road fell running style shoe, which tended to have much harder nobbled soles and a distinct lack of cushioning. They were still classified as trail shoes but were more like road shoes with more protruded grip on the soles. In the end the type of shoe to buy was decided after yet another conversation with Bill. According to the sage, fell shoes are great if you are off-road for the whole event but they can be pretty uncomfortable for any serious distances on harder ground. Given that the Green Man had a few lengthy sections of road particularly near the end, the softer hybrid shoe seemed to be a good all-rounder. As a final decider, the Kanadia were dirt cheap.

Training during the working day was almost always going to mean having somebody else to run with. As well as Bear who I worked with, several other members of our small department were also runners, as well as a handful of other people around the business in various departments. With the Bath Half Marathon also coming up in the spring, and working for a business located in Bath, there was no shortage of people keen to get out and run, which meant finding training partners was easy. Running in a group though comes with its own challenges as you do have to try to balance the speed and effort for the mixed abilities of all, which sometimes isn't possible, however after a few sessions natural groups tend to form and you end up with people of comparable abilities to run with.

Lunchtime runs were always going to be constrained by the hour time limit imposed upon us, so deciding to make the most out of that hour, a plan was devised to fit in as many off-road runs as we could, as well as spending time building strength with a hill running challenge. As a city Bath may be small and beautiful but it is also very hilly, with the main part of town being at the bottom of a valley, surrounded by hills most ways you turn. This proved opportunistic for hill running and Bear meticulously devised a chart of twelve hills, each graded and colour-coded by length and difficulty and he designed a nice little chart with places for cup stickers for each hill achieved. Without realising it we had reduced hill training to the level of a child's behaviour sticker chart. There was however no bag of Haribo or other treat in store for those completing all the hills. As well as the hills, we mapped routes along the canal towpath, cycletrack sections and through as many parks as we could find, that kept us off the main roads and away from traffic. There weren't huge numbers of routes as we were constrained by time, but with the combination of some variety and the ability to compare performance over the same route we had enough to work with.

It was on the first Monday in October, the day after the Bristol Half Marathon that I set out on my first proper lunchtime training run. I had mapped a route which ran alongside the Kennet and Avon Canal before turning off, under the main Bath to London railway line, over a bridge spanning the River Avon and back through a woodland footpath. It was a nice run and although my legs felt slightly heavy from the day before I managed what felt like a steady pace. Having not run the route before I wasn't actually sure where it led, so when I came across a path leading out to a car park I had to make a quick call on whether to jump off or to carry on. However, intent with getting as many off-road miles in as I could I carried on through the undergrowth, where I stumbled across an old guy sat in a bushy alcove drinking from a three-litre bottle of cider. As I ran by I looked at him and he looked back at me with a slightly confused look on his face but said nothing. About four-hundred metres later however, the path I was following came to an abrupt end. Unless I could scale a ten-foot wall, or swim across the river, my only choice was to double back on myself to the car park I spotted earlier. So turning around I jogged slowly back past the cider drinker and stating the obvious fact that we now both knew to be true: *"Dead end that way then"*, *"Yep"* came his simple reply. On the plus side at least I'd covered an extra half mile. Following the path out of the woods and into a Morrisons car park, I ran out onto the London Road and back to work through a park and along the River Avon. A nice little four mile loop, that we would come to use regularly, with the exception of not bothering to call on the tramp again.

A few days later I had arranged to run into work, meeting up with Bear along the way. Leaving home at six-thirty it was still dark, and seeing as we were approaching autumn with the sun not rising early, I wore another of my recent birthday gifts – an LED headtorch. Whilst it was pretty bright, running on main roads with streetlights still on it didn't prove very useful. I ran about three miles from my house to Keynsham to meet up with Bear, a route that I could've taken through a small wood near my house, but seeing as it was pitch black at the time I decided it would be a little too creepy for me (even with the headtorch) given that I'm not well known for my love of the dark. After meeting up we ran down the A4 into Saltford before dropping down onto the cycletrack into Bath, in the end covering about twelve miles. It was a slow and steady run but a good way to build the miles up. It would be runs like these to and from work, that wouldn't get too much in the way of everything else, that would allow us to build our weekly mileage up.

The following Friday Bear and I had decided to run a double header and run both into work and home again. Given that the full distance would be a bit too much of a jump, we decided to both drive to Avon Valley Railway in Bitton and run in from there. This was a journey of seven miles, which at both ends of the day added together would give us a nice round fourteen. The run in was uneventful but after working a full day the idea of running another seven miles home again seemed a little insane. We donned our still sweaty wet kit (note to self – bring spare kit if running a double in the future) and set off back along the cycletrack towards Bitton. The first couple of miles were tough and we both questioned if we had maybe been a touch unrealistic, a couple of miles in however it was as if a switch had been flipped. We gained a new wind and ran back to our cars as if it was the first run of the day. It was a very satisfying feeling.

The following weekend was lost due to my wife working, but thinking outside of the box and determined to get a run in, I decided to try to get out and do what I could with my two kids riding their bikes alongside me. Whilst this sounds like a great idea in terms of having a pacing team, pushing and encouraging me, I should state that they were only seven and nine years old and weren't really pacing material, especially seeing as Louis, the youngest of the two had only just learnt to ride his bike without stabilisers. I enticed them with the promise of seeing a big tunnel and without really telling them how far away it was. Having sold my idea (something about the promise of sweets probably swung it), we set out from Warmley Station heading towards Bristol and the Staple Hill Tunnel, which at about four-hundred metres in length is a pretty dark and dingy place. Overall I was surprised by how well they rode, even though they couldn't keep a steady pace. With one of the only hills on the entire path to cycle up, Louis powered up it admirably with his wobbly and weaving stabiliser-less pedalling and carried on to the entrance to the tunnel. As expected, once we got there they were less than impressed by the superb feat of civil engineering and we more or less turned straight around and headed back. It was at a brief respite stop at the remains of Mangotsfield Station on the way back when I noticed the front tyre on Louis' bike was a lot softer than when we started. A puncture? I could do without that. So off we went quickly, me encouraging Louis to ride as fast as he could to get back to the car before it went completely flat and I would have to carry it back walking. As luck would have it we made it back to Warmley with the tyre squidging all over the place. Overall a mild success of a Sunday afternoon: one puncture, two bags of sweets and five more miles in the bank – albeit very slow ones.

It was the following Friday that we officially started the hill challenge. During a lunchtime run, me, Bear and another work runner, Scott, ventured out to tackle the first couple of hills. Scott Martin wasn't a dedicated runner but was a pretty fit individual who tended to go to the gym before work most days. With past running experiences such as the Bath Half Marathon as well as a number of triathlons he was certainly a decent runner, but with spending more time in the gym pushing weights working his upper body than lower he did have the appearance of Mr Rush from the Mr Men series of books (somewhat triangular). His self-admitted chicken legs did well to power him around local races in very respectable times, but running wasn't really his first love. He was of course still significantly slimmer and fitter (not to mention younger) than me.

The run took in a hike up the Wells Road and then the Wellsway, which was a slow mountain of a road heading out of Bath; up as far as the Midford turn-off then loop back down through Foxhill towards the centre again, before taking a minor detour to run up Rosemount Lane. With a quaint sounding name, you might think that Rosemount was a pretty little hill with flowers all up the side to look at as you slowly jogged up it. You would be wrong. The first thing that would give it away would be the 25% sign at the bottom. Whilst it is only around two-hundred and fifty metres from top to bottom, boy is it tough. In a stark contrast from the slow plodding up the long mellow Wellsway, Rosemount Lane is a short sharp shock. If Wellsway was a cup of English breakfast tea, then Rosemount would be a shot of Absinth. Coming as it did at the end of a four mile run it was never going to be a breeze, but we all got up it with a touch of swearing and sweating. There aren't many hills you get to the top of and have to sit down but this is one of those few, certainly at this point in time. The thing is when you are fit you can choose to have an easy run and take it steady, when you are unfit there is no such thing as an easy run. Everything is too far or too fast. Getting to that point of fitness would be a key point in my training however I certainly wasn't there yet. We jogged back to the office with two hills in the bank and two stickers on the chart. Like a group of toddlers who've just been given smiley faces for weeing on the potty, we were overjoyed.

The start of the third week of October I managed to get back to a long weekend run and managed to plod my way around without an issue. I ran for the first time with another of my birthday presents, a 10 litre Deuter Speedlite backpack (oh yes, I had an exciting birthday that year), which I would be running the Green Man with, loaded with water and food. Inside the backpack was a two litre drinks bladder, with a tube which came out the top of the bag so you can hydrate on the move – very important for ultras where you would be out for hours at a time. Monday saw Bear, Scott and I collect another two stickers by conquering both Lyncombe Hill and Entry Hill with some ease during our lunch. Then on a sticker roll, Tuesday saw the third hill of the week, running up Shakespeare Avenue to Alexandra Park, which offers probably the best view over Bath bar none. This time it was me and Scott, together with Tim (with whom I ran the Bristol Half Marathon) and another office runner Rebecca Rogers. Rebecca was a natural runner and one of those annoying people who made it look easy. Despite her diminutive stature, coming in at around five foot three, she had all the speed of somebody with legs twice as long and yet still managed to make it look effortless. Running with her trademark earphones in just one ear so as to only be partly rude whilst running in a group, she joined us during some of our lunchtime runs (so long as it wasn't raining and she didn't get her hair wet), as she was running the Bath Half Marathon which was the same weekend as the ultra. For the first time during our lunchtime sessions somebody was pushing the pace on the flats – although she would never admit to it. All I know is that Scott and I were blowing like an old exhaust trying to keep up with her. What I had found was now I had started to wear the heart rate monitor, it was proving difficult to moderate my heart rate when running with others. Trying to keep pace with somebody else, fast or slow caused issues with the training zones I was supposed to be working within. Something I would need to work on if I was going to get the most from the training.

The next day I decided to run by myself and try to regulate my pace by my heart rate alone, tackling another one of the hills on the sheet – Lansdown Road. I had mapped out a route taking in the hill and looping back through some woods, so I got a hill and some off-road work in one run. Running up to Lansdown I kept my pace slow as I was watching my heart rate, trying to keep it in the 140–169bpm range as specified by Jonathan in his report. What I found was that running by heart rate meant I was running up the hill slower than I would normally, hence I got to the top with less exertion than I would have done if I wasn't running within the constraints of the heart rate training zones. Once at the top of the hill I turned and ran back down to Bath through Primrose Hill Community Woodland, which was seriously muddy, down into Weston following the Cotswold Way footpath into town and back into work. Three weeks into training and weight loss and I was starting to notice a difference. Running was getting easier and my clothes were starting to feel looser. It was a good feeling, a sense of progress. With North Road, another hill conquered, running with Scott, Tim and Rebecca on the Friday, the week was also proving very fruitful for sticker collecting.

The final week of October saw another long Sunday run followed by lunchtime runs every day bar Friday, together with running into work on Wednesday. It was a pretty high mileage week but a successful one. Feeling good on Wednesday morning I decided to run into work by myself following the ten miles from my house and along the Bitton to Bath cycletrack. Worryingly my right knee started to feel a bit funny as I left home, almost like it was going to give out on me. As runners do, I just carried on and hoped it would just go away. It got worse before it got better, but about three miles in as I came up on Bitton it just went away. It was a bit of a concern, although could possibly be nothing more than a touch of overtraining. I ran on following my heart rate monitor trying to keep my BPM in somewhere in the 150 range, which was the middle of the zone I should be training in. What I found was that it was more difficult than I thought as when I was running at what I thought was a steady pace I found my heart rate too low, so I picked up the pace again and again until my heart was turning over at 155bpm, but I

him and the issues I had with my gluteus medius locking up and having so many cascading problems. Once I got up on the table on my side and stuck my right leg up in the air, he pushed it straight back down with almost no effort or resistance. I just couldn't hold him off at all. I turned over and we tested my left leg and I could hold off his strongest push. It was incredible to see the difference. Dave's diagnosis was tightened glutetus medius – a classic overtraining injury, hopefully we had caught it early.

Diagnosis complete, Dave started with a bit of loosening up of the offending muscles. Five minutes kneading and pushing later and we did a re-test of the glute strength. This time it was like somebody had swapped my leg with somebody else's. There was no way he was pushing it down again. It was amazing what a bit of manipulation in the right place could do. He followed up with some iliotibial band (ITB) loosening and some painful kneading, but forty-five minutes later and he's all done and I have both legs back in full action. He gave me some exercises and stretches and said the knee pain would fade away. Time would tell.

7. Slogging it Out

"They shall grow not old, as we that are left grow old:
Age shall not weary them, nor the years condemn.
At the going down of the sun and in the morning,
We will remember them." – **Laurence Binyon**

I always think that any town that starts with the word Chipping just sounds a bit twee from the off and I don't think Chipping Sodbury lets my theory down. A small market town to the north of Bristol (Chipping literally translates from Old English as market) it has all the hallmarks of a nice middle-class rural town where not much really happens. That is until Remembrance Sunday each November when the population of the town increases by around a fifth thanks to the annual mud-fest that is the Easy Runner Sodbury Slog. According to the website *"The Sodbury Slog is quite simply not for the faint-hearted! Forget roads – they're for wimps – this was a lung-busting, trainer-ruining, hill-climbing, multi-terrain challenge held over and through some of South Gloucestershire's most stunning countryside."* The race was a multi-terrain event, run over roughly nine miles and organised by Bitton Road Runners under the directorship of Gordon Robbins. It was a race that had an excellent reputation and as soon as entries opened each year it sold out in a matter of weeks. A reflection of how well the event was put together and how much fun it was. Don't get me wrong this was a serious event that attracted serious runners from all over the UK and further afield, many of whom came back time and again to take on the mud. But it was also a race for all abilities in which you couldn't help but smile.

The first race over a similar course was run in 1990 and was originally called the Beagle Bash, with the name changing to The Sodbury Slog in 1999. Much of the race takes place on private land and local farmer John Ludlow, who was an active member of the Rotary Club of Chipping Sodbury, obtains the necessary landowner permission for the race to go ahead. Without the support of the landowners the race could not take place. Members of Bitton Road Runners, the Rotary Club and the local community all help marshal the event each year and in return over £2 per entrant is donated to local charities and the community, which is distributed by the Rotary Club of Chipping Sodbury.

Given the off-road nature of the event I decided it would make a great training run for the Green Man. Talking to Gordon I managed to secure five places and signed up Bear, Tim, Scott, Scott's girlfriend Gina and me. Also joining us was a former Bitton member I knew well, Burnie (whose actual name was Ant, not that anyone ever used it). The plan on the day was to all try and run together (although not Gina as she drank far too much wine at a wedding reception most of us attended the night before, where because we were running I bought one of the most boring round of drinks ever – a lemonade, two cokes, an orange juice and half a lager). All very sober (except Gina) we rolled up at Chipping Sodbury School around ten o'clock, collected our numbers and race chips and stood around discussing tactics. Having actually run the race some five times before I was an old hand at it, and with the exception of Burnie who had also run it a couple of times, nobody else really knew what to expect. For the unwary there is always a short video on the event website[*] showing what you can expect, starring a slightly chubby yours truly. In 2006 I ran the race as part of a feature for the BBC One series *Inside Out West*. The idea was to run with local television weatherman Richard Angwin, showing why the race had such a good reputation. What

---

[*] You can watch the video at http://www.facebook.com/fm2gm

they got was me and Rich getting plastered in mud and having a blast. I ran carrying a BBC issue camera, which because it got so muddy, almost none of the footage from it could be used. Luckily there were other cameramen around the route to capture the fun. Obviously we didn't run a very fast time that year, stopping to talk to cameramen along the way will always do that but that's not why we did it anyway.

The thing is with the Slog, to run a good time there are only two things you need know: 1) tie your shoes on pretty bloody tight – once they get sucked off in a bog you're going to struggle to find them and 2) get out fast – like Road Runner fast. The first mile of the race is actually on tarmac, so getting that first mile covered as quickly as possible allows you to get as far up the field of runners as you can. Why? Well, mostly because the mud is a lot less churned up and more solid when only one hundred people have been through it as opposed to one thousand.

Being held on Remembrance Sunday the race was always preceded by the exhortation, two minutes silence and playing of the Last Post. In all the years I had run the event I always found this quite emotional. To have over a thousand runners and supporters all milling around chatting to suddenly go so silent you could hear a pin drop, followed by the bugle player is equally both chilling and moving. It really does make you stop and think, which is exactly what it is designed to do, think and remember.

After the bugle has played and the applause has gone around everyone moves out of the school grounds en masse onto the road outside ready for the starting klaxon. We were all grouped together and ready to run, slowly pushing our way down the grass embankment to get closer to the front when the horn sounded and we were off.

The weight loss had been going pretty well and I was now 15st 1lb and my fitness had noticeably improved along with it. Given all of that I decided to set myself two goals for the day. The first was simply to run my fastest Slog ever and the second was to beat Scott. Seeing as he was over ten years younger than me and significantly fitter overall, it would be a great morale boost to finish ahead of him. The funny thing is I never consider myself a competitive person, unless that is I think I actually have a chance of winning then I go at it flying. This was one of those days. As its name suggests though the race isn't exactly short and sweet and I really wanted us to run the bulk of it together, so I decided it was a case of picking my moment carefully.

We shot off down Bowling Road heading into Chipping Sodbury town centre, before turning off left onto the Wickwar road. As we clocked the first mile my GPS watch beeped and I looked down to see it recorded as 7 minutes 20 seconds, which while not the fastest mile ever recorded it was a damn sight faster than anything I'd run recently. No wonder I was blowing already, but we were still warming into it and that would be time in the bank. I would be able to catch my breath once we hit the mud and naturally slowed down. Burnie, Scott and I were all still together and looking back I saw Bear not too far behind. We had already lost Tim. Rounding the corner, past the golf club we stepped onto the first of the off-road sections and it was wet and very muddy. Every step saw your foot sink a little and slip a little more. I was wearing the Adidas Kanadia which were better than road shoes on this terrain but you couldn't exactly say they were grippy. Hitting the mud, Bear had trouble keeping his footing and started to slow down behind us. I put it down to him being so tall and having a higher centre of gravity that balancing on a slippery surface was tricky. He didn't seem able to keep the same pace as us and at one point we did slow to see if he could catch us up, but we'd already lost sight of him. Tim however failed rule one of the Slog handbook and had neglected to tie his laces tight enough and lost a shoe very early on, paying the price in time trying to find it in the quagmire, which luckily he did. There have been cases in previous years where runners have lost shoes early on in the race and have made the executive decision to go on without them. At some time in the far future an archaeologist is probably going to have a very interesting find that could take some explaining.

As the race wore on we just kept going. Being up near the front of the pack the going was still good and when we came to obstacles such as hay bales and the sheep dip there were no queues to hold us up. We were making good progress ploughing through the turned fields, up the hills, through woods and through the Iron Age hill fort. Every time we hit a short stretch of tarmac on a country lane we would run whilst stamping our feet to try and break off the excess mud as it only added unwanted ballast to each leg. After the shame of not wearing my club vest at the Bristol Half Marathon some six weeks previous, I wore it with pride that day given that my slightly smaller frame didn't stretch the seams to breaking point and I'm glad I did. The support from the race marshals at the Slog is always second to none and they really help get people around but when so many of them were fellow Bitton club members who knew me it meant there was great encouragement at almost every corner. Scott thought it was comical the amount of people who cheered me on by my name and likened it to running with a celebrity. But he was the one who deserved the recognition that day. He pushed the three of us pretty hard most of the way round and I would say he was the one setting the pace. Had I not ran with him I don't think I would have run anywhere near as well that day. In all the years I've ran the Slog I'd never actually managed to run the whole way around before, this was something of a first. Despite initially having planned to race hard and beat Scott to the finish, having stayed together all the way around I had thought it would be more appropriate that we crossed the line together, holding hands or something. That was until we entered into the school grounds and Burnie suggested a sprint finish. As soon as I heard the cry I went, I didn't stop to question the others for a heartbeat, nor did I look back to see where they were – I just bolted. I ran flat out around the building weaving in and out of other runners, around the corner to see not the finish but another building. I kept it going and pushed on, thinking the end was just in my grasp, I just had to hold on a little longer but rounding the next corner I still didn't see the finishing arch, just another building. It was like running on Groundhog Day. Without looking back I yelped to those chasing me down that I fear I may have gone too early but I kept pushing. If I was tiring, then so must they be. Then around the next corner finally was the glorious finish line. As I crossed the line I was so engrossed with winning I even forgot to stop my watch. I was excited to the point that you would have thought that I had won the whole race. Being fair, the real winner out of the three of us that day was Scott (although technically history will record it as being me). Without his stamina pulling us all the way around I would have given in and walked the same places I usually did in the Slog and been at least five minutes down. In the end I finished in 1 hour 19 minutes, which was my fastest Slog time ever, placing me third home for the club (although to be fair many of the better club runners were busy marshalling the route).

Overall it was quite simply the best Slog I had ever run. I thought that maybe it was a slightly quicker course this time around, as it does vary slightly year on year, although looking at the results the winning time was pretty much as it had been in previous years so I think it was fair to say it was probably comparable.

As our first real off-road jaunt it had been a success. Bear finished just ten minutes behind Scott, Burnie and I and almost enjoyed it. If anything it highlighted to him how much tougher off-road running really was and that he needed to work on his mud-gripping skills. Tim finished less than a minute behind Bear and Gina rolled over the line feeling less queasy than she started in a highly commendable

8. Training Diary: November

"Motivation is what gets you started. Habit is what keeps you going."
– Jim Ryun

Total Miles Run: 126.75
Highest Weekly Total: 45.75
Weekly Average: 28.62

One whole month into training and weight loss, and everything was going reasonably well. I still had the niggling knee problem but hopefully the work that Dave had done and stretches he'd given me were going to do the trick. Being an all or nothing person my resolve had become a fortress against cakes, double lunches, needless eating and of course beer, all of which, combined with the running, had brought my weight down by a whole stone by the start of November. It was good going and I was certainly starting to notice the difference in my training as well as my clothes. I read one statistic suggesting each pound of body fat lost can equate to an improvement of around two seconds per mile in pace. Throw some extra training in there too and you're only going to be getting faster and stronger.

It was Guy Fawkes Night and I was invited to a family barbeque at my sister's house, so as a small treat I decided to buy myself a four pack of 330ml bottles of Heineken. I've always thought it's important to not completely abstain from anything or you are bound to fail, but just learn to moderate it. Moderation evidently being the one thing I had always failed miserably at in the past. But having gone from drinking probably four 500ml cans of beer four or five nights a week, dropping down to four small bottles in one month didn't seem like I was going overboard. Was I looking forward to sipping on the cold crisp golden nectar in those bottles? Yes and no. I was looking forward to it because I hadn't had any beer for a month but on the flipside the little health angel in my head was telling me not to give in. I didn't see it as giving in though, I saw it as moderation. I guess it all depends upon perspective. I think the important thing to realise when trying to learn to moderate is that you aren't actually giving anything up. You are just swapping one thing you like for another, with the other in this case being better health and fitness. Did I like beer? Hell yeah! But did I also want to be fitter and healthier? Yes again and at this point in time I wanted the latter more than the former. So, slightly frothing at the mouth and with some excitement I cracked open the first bottle and took a small sip. It was like heaven had run a tap into my mouth. The taste was wonderful, and the funny thing was I could actually taste it. When you drink all the time it becomes habitual and you lose the ability to really taste any of it, it just becomes fluid. This though was gorgeous all the way to the bottom of the little green bottle. However when I opened and started on the second bottle that golden flavour had already gone and taken the magic with it. I just didn't enjoy it the same way as the first. With the initial desire sated, it seemed the rest weren't really required. Obviously I still drank all four, I'm not that good. I wasn't however in a rush to have any more.

As we were now well into winter the weather had turned for the worse and it appeared to be raining a lot of the time. This though was irrelevant to my training as I had come to live by the Phil mantra: *"once you're wet, you're wet"*. And anyway, if you're training for an event, how do you know it's not going to be raining on that day?

On the first Sunday of the month I had arranged to run ten miles with Burnie, keeping the distance down as my knee was still playing up and the last thing I wanted was to make it worse now. As dedicated as I am to a goal, sometimes you really have to question yourself and this morning was one of those times. With a sore knee, driving rain, strong winds and even a touch of snow towards the end, we ploughed a loop around Kingswood, Warmley and Shortwood. It wasn't fun and I was certainly glad to get home that morning. A couple of days later at work, running with Rebecca and another good friend and work colleague Jon, we decided to try and tackle one of the biggest remaining challenges on the sticker chart, Bathwick Hill. Jon Westlake was one of my oldest friends having both started work in the same place on the same week, back in 1999. Over the years we had ran together, worked together, gone to beer festivals together and I was even best man at his wedding. We got on so well because we had very much the same interests and attitude. Jon's running career however had been intermittent over the years but he was very capable when he put his mind to it. We had ran the Paris Half Marathon and a number of 10K races together over the years and now we were working together again, he had been coaxed back into running given most of our team were. Heading out of the office we ran out towards the A36 until we came to the bottom of Bathwick Hill where the challenge began. Bathwick was one of the red hills on the chart, given it was both long and steep. It was just over one mile to climb and with a gradient steep enough to knock the wind out of you before you got even halfway up. I was wearing my heart rate monitor and was keen to get to the top keeping my beats per minute (BPM) in the correct training range, so ran with one eye on it as we climbed. Starting off together, Rebecca kept pace with my longer strides with ease, almost floating up the hill, with Jon close behind. About halfway up the hill it appeared to level out a touch giving you a false sense of hope that you have finished, whereas it in fact climbs more steeply again before reaching the top. From about the halfway point I slowly pulled away and edged my

jogged slowly alongside encouraging him to the finish. At the top we high-fived our double achievement, only a month ago we would flag trying to make it up one of those hills, now here we were having conquered not just one of the toughest hills on the chart, but two in one run. When we got back to the office and collected our two stickers, the others just shook their head. From that one lunchtime session the bar had now been raised. We had proved that two hills in one session was possible. The following day I set out again with Tim, Bear, Scott and Jon and again ran two hills during one lunch, a feat which everybody pulled off. Double was the new normal.

The following Friday I was planning on having a rest day. My knee had started to feel better and hadn't been troubling me, however it had been a pretty high mileage week so didn't want to push my luck. However when I was asked if I wanted to get a few slow miles in over lunch I thought why not. The plan was to run up the Wellsway so a few others could gain their stickers. By this time a good dozen others in the company had now taken on the hill challenge, together with a group training for the Bath Half Marathon. Bear had suggested that we put in a team of runners, raising money for the Forever Friends appeal at the Royal United Hospital (RUH) in Bath. The team was made up of a mixture of people, many who had never run before and liked the idea of taking on the half marathon. Everyone had their own reasons for taking on the challenge but for one girl it was purely about weight loss and fitness and for good reason. Fay Ellis worked in a different department to us and was good friends with Scott. She wasn't a tall girl, somewhere around five foot two, but was definitely a larger lady. In her own words she was a *"short fat hobbit with a large personality"*. To her, the idea of running a half marathon seemed like a pipe dream. She was unfit and overweight, something she had always struggled with. However, with a positive disposition and the encouragement and help of Scott, Bear and I, she decided to take on the challenge in a very familiar bid to lose

really swollen or bruised and the pain seemed to have receded. It was however a stark warning of the fine line between fitness and injury. It could've so easily been a broken ankle up there on that path and the whole challenge would have been completely out of the window. Even a free helicopter ride wouldn't have made up for that.

The following day with my ankle seemingly recovered, I set out on my own on my first recce of the Community Forest Path. This is what it was all about and today was going to be my first taste of what was to come. A section of the path passed through Warmley which was close to my house, so I drove there and parked up, planning a slow looping route of about eleven or twelve miles. Armed with my OS map tucked in my bag (complete with nice pink line drawn over the path) I set off from Warmley Station car park towards Winterbourne. But after a couple of hundred metres I reached some woods and the path split into two. I was stumped already, failing at the very first choice. I got the map out and consulted, opting for the path to the right and ran on. If this was indicative of the rest of the route it was going to be a long morning. The path ran on through Warmley Forest up towards Siston Common, through some fields and ending up at Shortwood. The route was pretty boggy and it didn't take long to get seriously wet and muddy. It was however all pretty familiar territory as it was my side of town; however as I was leaving Shortwood I made my first error. Looking for the footpath sign I followed the wrong sign and ended up in a big field running around looking for a way out. Walking round the field looking for a stile I decided to get my phone out, turn the GPS on and look at Google Maps. What a waste of time that was. It might be great on roads but all it told me now was that I was stood in the middle of a field in Shortwood. I didn't need GPS to tell me that. I decided the best thing to do would be to trace my footsteps back to my last known good point and consult the OS map properly. It was only as I got back to the stile I'd just come over that I saw the Community

Forest Footpath sign on a post – pointing in the other direction. Back on the right path I ran across a large field full of sheep, passed through a kissing gate and onto a tarmac lane which led me down to somebody's driveway. Surely this couldn't be right. Looking around again behind me I saw a footpath sign pointing into the field next to the house, so I went through the kissing gate and ran down over the field. It took me five minutes to realise that there wasn't actually a way out in the direction I needed to go. Fail two. So once again I turned around and went back to the last known point and looked again. Staring at the driveway to the house in front of me I saw the remnants of a Community Forest Path sticker on a post pointing towards the house. Suddenly I remembered one of Bill's golden nuggets of information. He told us that at one point on the path it looked as if you were going into somebody's house but at the last-minute the path went around it. The trouble was I couldn't remember where on the route that was, but I guessed this could be it. So acting dead casual, looking like I was a postman going to deliver the mail and hoping that the quiet isolated house in the woods didn't belong to some lunatic runner murderer, I jogged cautiously down the driveway towards the house. Then, just before I reached the front door, I clocked a footpath sign directing me through a tiny gap in a fence and around to the right of the house. Quickly I followed the sign through the fence and down a footpath, taking me into some woods heading away from the house. I ran on without looking back to see if 'mother' was watching at me out of a bedroom window. The muddy path continued on around a particularly unattractive and stinky landfill site and ended up on a stretch of tarmac cycletrack heading away from Emersons Green. From there it seemed fairly straightforward. Through a few fields, under the M4 motorway, through some more woods ending up in Kendleshire. Thanks to the rain, most of the fields were at least shin deep in mud and water, which made for very slow and dirty progress. For some reason

9. Up Above the Streets and Houses

"Racing is the fun part; it's the reward of all the hard work."
– **Kara Goucher**

The city of Bath is a world heritage site, famed for its iconic Roman baths, splendid Palladian architecture and distinct lack of either an Aldi or Lidl store. Whilst it can be nice traipsing around the sights with the millions of other tourists, it is possible to get a great view of the city from the hills above, in particular from the National Trust Bath Skyline walk. The path is a rural loop of roughly six miles that takes you through woodland, hidden valleys and scenic landscape gardens. More importantly it offers an unrivalled elevated view over the city, so long as you're not head down racing around it ankle deep in mud in the wettest depths of winter.

As the name suggested the Skyline 10K series was a collection of four trail races put on by Relish Running Races that took place on and around part of the National Trust footpath high above the city. Running from November through February each year, they offered runners frost, rain and mud over two variants of the route used alternately through the series. Seeing as how they were off-road in nature and how I was trying to get in as much multi-terrain experience as I could over the winter months, I decided it would be fun to tackle the December event. In the office Jon had already signed himself up to run the entire series, so a brief email and some discussion later a group of six hardy souls, including Scott, Fay and myself decided to run the Skyline as a bit of pre-Christmas off-road fun. Following on from the success of the Slog the previous month and a bit of off-road running at lunchtime Scott and I were developing our mud legs pretty well. However, whereas at the Slog Scott had set the pace, I was confident I had moved on over the last few weeks and decided it was time to run my own race – and obviously finish first. I found as my fitness was developing and I was becoming stronger, my sense of competition was also growing, which if nothing else just made for a more fun and challenging race. I knew that Scott would likely be out to level my Slog victory and that Jon's competitive spirit would drive him into the ground to try and beat us both but I was pretty sure I could hold them both at bay. I was going to go out like a train – albeit a train that ran well on mud.

The base for the event was the University of Bath Sports Training Village, the very same place I had attended the Human Performance Centre a couple of months previous and ran myself to exhaustion on the treadmill. With registration and number collection inside the main building on the morning, the event itself took place on a field adjacent to the main building, with a low-key gazebo setup for finishers and a start and finish area marked out with tape. Being winter nobody was particularly keen to strip down to race gear until the very last-minute, so the playing field became a warm up area for a wealth of fully-dressed runners all biding their time until the off. The flat grassy playing field gave nothing away as to how tough the route would be. It was a two-lap race, with a 5K running alongside, which meant you would need to be pretty careful who you tried keeping pace with. There can be nothing worse in a race than killing yourself trying to stick on somebody's shoulder all the way around only to see them peel off and finish halfway leaving you broken and dispirited with a lap still to go. It had been quite some time since I had raced over this distance and really wasn't sure what sort of time to expect, especially given the unknown element of the course. I figured to myself that at least if nothing else the second lap

an undulating muddy field that eventually took us down deep into the woods. This is where the going underfoot got really soft. It was a real trail with rocks and roots all over the place. The racing pack was still somewhat together which caused a bit of an issue for a troupe of Sunday morning hikers coming the other way along the footpath. Whilst everyone had an equal right of way on the path, there was no way any of the runners were going to stop to let Brian and Lesley pass by with their hiking poles and pockets full of Kendal Mint Cake. With the route through the woods not being entirely clear I simply followed the runner in front on the assumption he knew where he was going. Luckily he did, or at least the guy in front of him did. Getting out from under the tree cover meant a short, steep, slippery climb which even when wearing trail shoes was difficult to gain any real traction on. Watching the people in front trying to get up it was like watching the Chuckle Brothers roller skating on custard. Had I not been in a race it would have been funny just to sit there and spectate. I decided that I would walk this section, which proved to be a pretty good idea. Getting to the top of Mud Mountain took us into yet more woodland, which was followed by another small hill. Finally back on flat ground I ran on, through a kissing gate and through a final field taking me back into the university grounds. As I turned the last corner and ran up the familiar straight towards the halfway point I checked my watch to see how I was doing for time. Seeing 25 minutes 58 seconds on the clock it was pretty obvious that my target time of 45 minutes was woefully adrift from reality. With a long flat straight behind me as I headed back up towards the halls, I looked back to see if Scott or Jon were close however still couldn't see either of them. Feeling pretty safe from being caught I eased up a little to allow myself to catch my breath slightly and ran on up behind the dormitory buildings once more. Like a car journey on the way home the sights of the course were familiar the second time around and the route passed by quicker than the first. Coming back through the woods, the field was much more strung out than the first time around and there was nobody visible in front of me and just one runner close behind. Even the hikers had gone. The first time around I just blindly followed everyone else, but now I wasn't sure I was still going the right way. I kept running in a straight line hoping to see some kind of sign. Were there signs? Arrows even? In my desperate bid to outrun Scott and Jon, I paid so little attention the first time around I didn't even know if there had been any marshals hiding out in the woods. Luckily every time I thought I was lost I saw a random bit of tape hanging from a tree, so I just followed that and the guy behind me bought it too. We would have been scuppered if we had discovered a new type of tree that grew red and white plastic tape. Once again we came across the climb to get out of the woods; only this time somewhere close to two hundred people had already made their way up it making it much tougher to climb. A rope here would have been handy – or some steps – but as it was all I had to help get myself up was the odd tree root and my hands. Once I got back up onto the top and into the fields it was just a case of finding my way back onto the university campus and running up the final straight to the finish. The runner who had been close behind me in the woods made his move past me and pushed on to the finish. I was pretty tired and happy to let him go, especially seeing as how it wasn't Scott or Jon. Crossing the line I stopped my GPS watch and took a look down, 53 minutes 58 seconds. Quite a way off my initial goal of 45 minutes, although given the final distance was closer to seven miles than six I'll take it – especially seeing as the winner (a super-slim guy clad in Royal Navy lycra) only ran a time of 45 minutes 30 seconds and I was twenty-eighth.

I walked over to the race gazebo and collected my goodie bag, Father Christmas medal and scoffed down a couple of mince pies that were there for the taking. I walked back to the side of the field where runners were still streaming in to wait for the others. First to

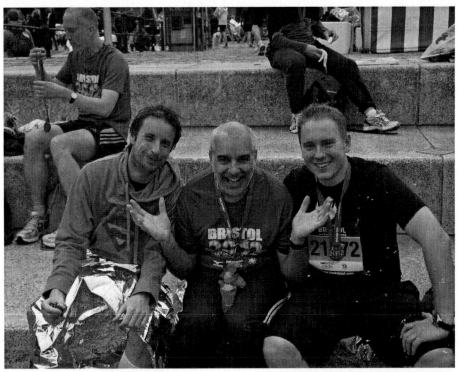

Bear, me and Tim at the end of the 2012 Bristol Half Marathon.

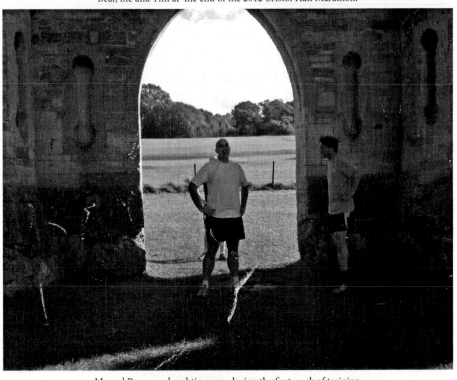

Me and Bear on a lunchtime run during the first week of training.

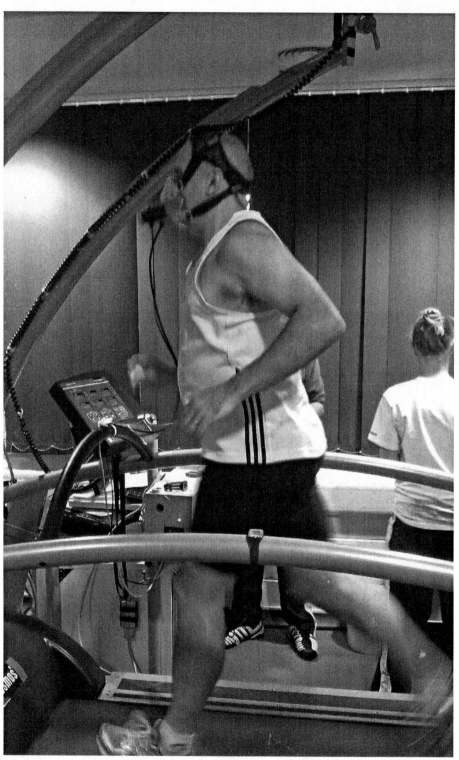

A fat man undergoing a first set of fitness tests at the University of Bath.

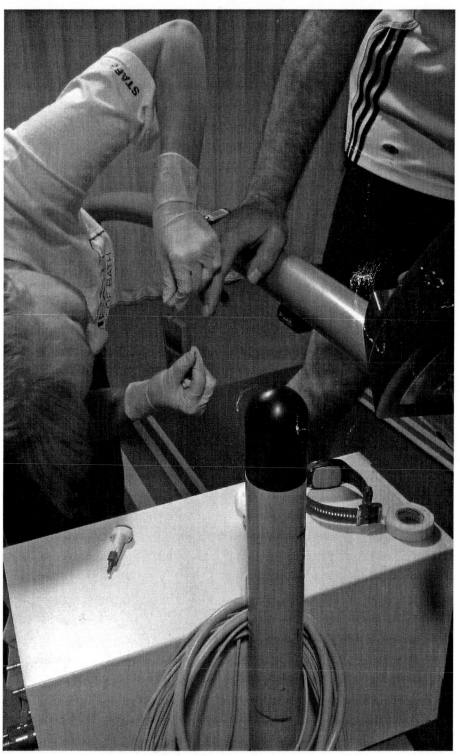
Having blood taken during the treadmill test to check lactate levels.

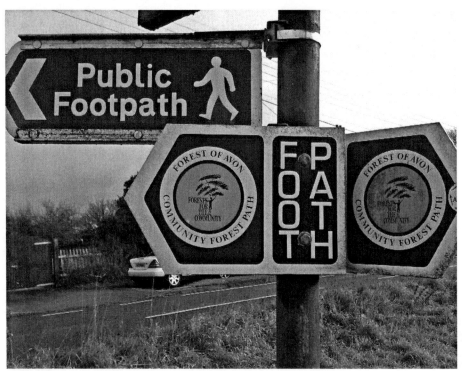

The Community Forest Path signs found during my first recce run.

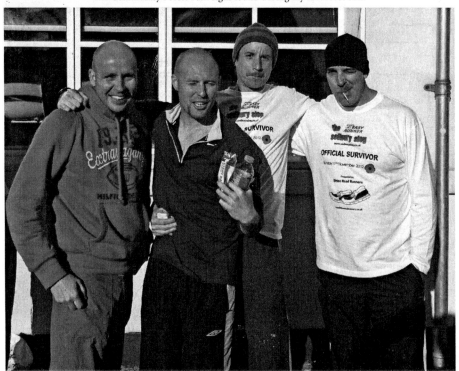

Burnie, Scott, Bear and me after running the 2012 Sodbury Slog.

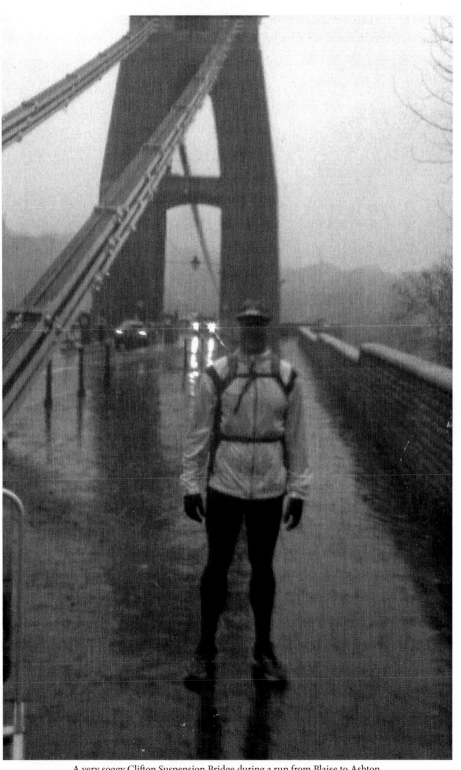

A very soggy Clifton Suspension Bridge during a run from Blaise to Ashton.

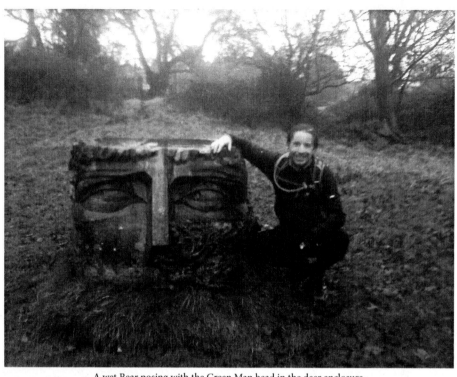

A wet Bear posing with the Green Man head in the deer enclosure.

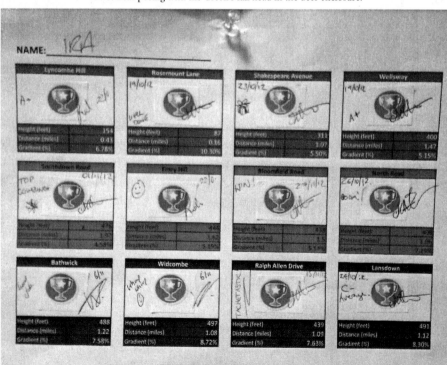

A successfully completed hill training chart complete with stickers.

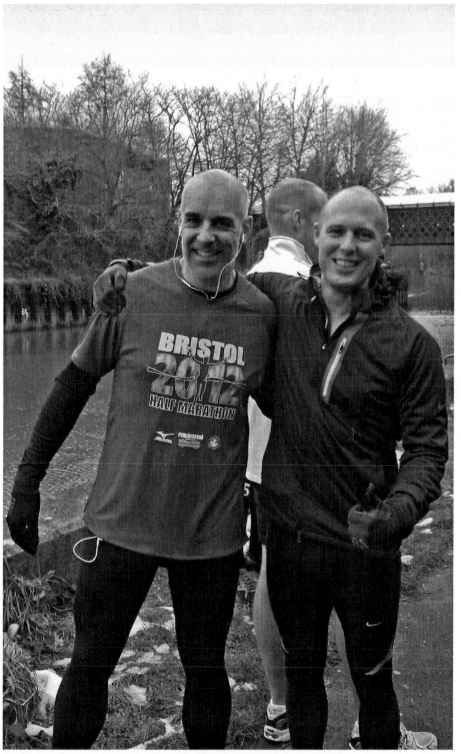

Me and Scott getting ready for another handicap challenge.

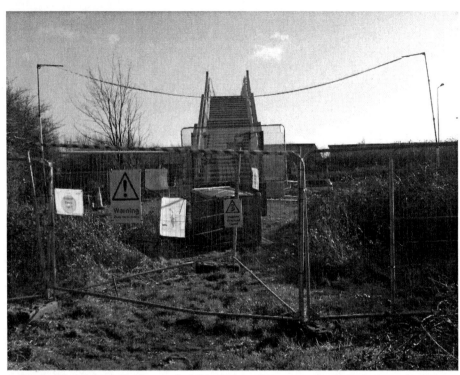
The closed bridge over the M5 in Patchway that we in no way climbed over.

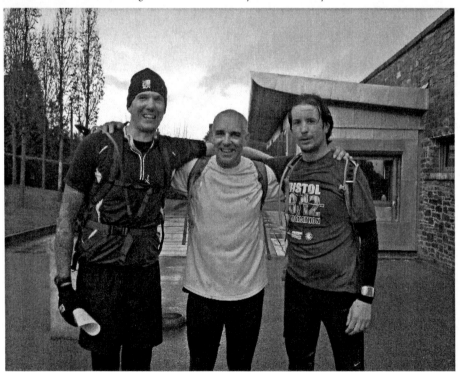
Guy, me and Bear after completing a twenty-three mile recce from Keynsham to Blaise.

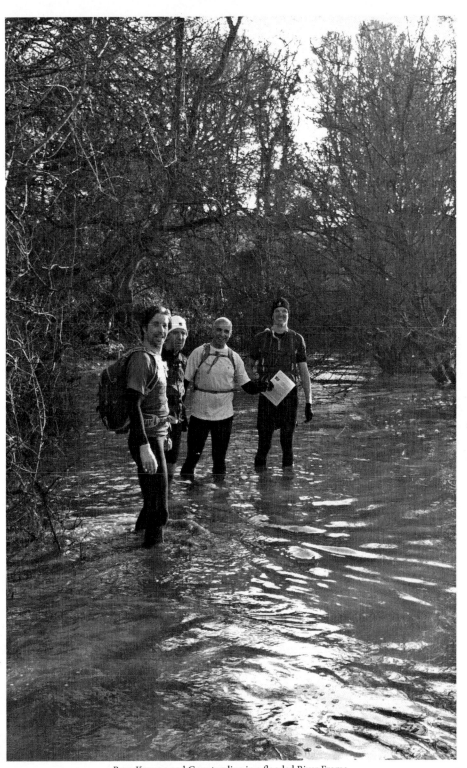

Bear, Kev, me and Guy standing in a flooded River Frome.

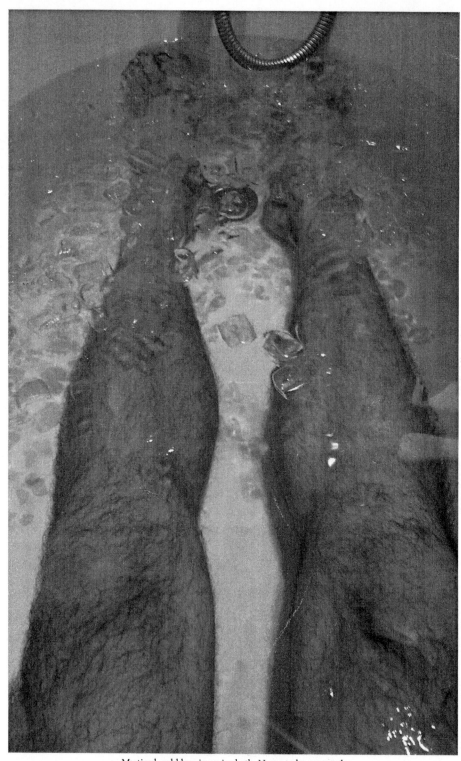

My tired, cold legs in an ice bath. Never to be repeated.

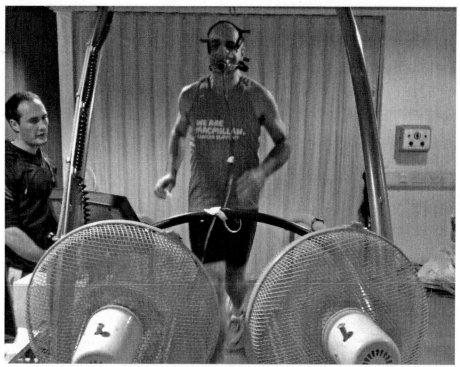

A much slimmer and fitter me at the second fitness test in February.

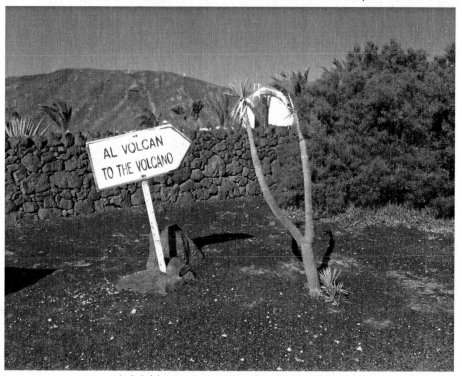

The helpful sign pointing to the volcano in Playa Blanca.

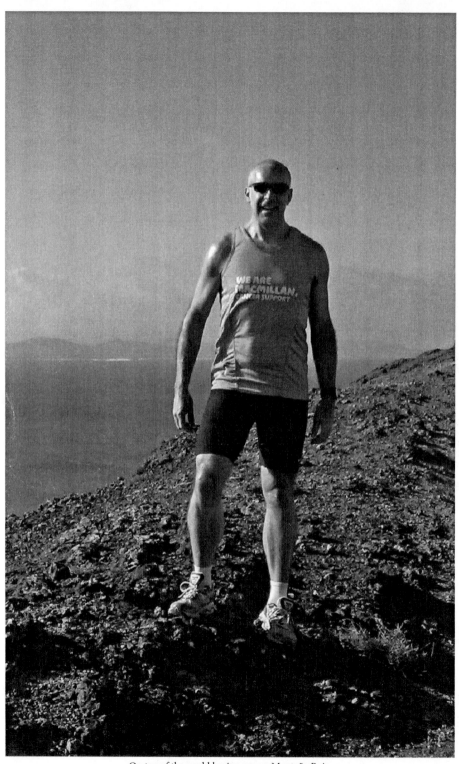

On top of the world having ran up Montaña Roja.

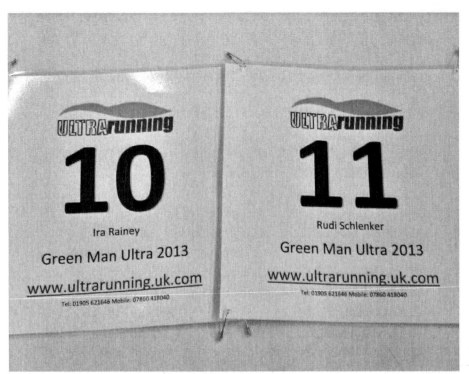

Race numbers collected and ready for the off.

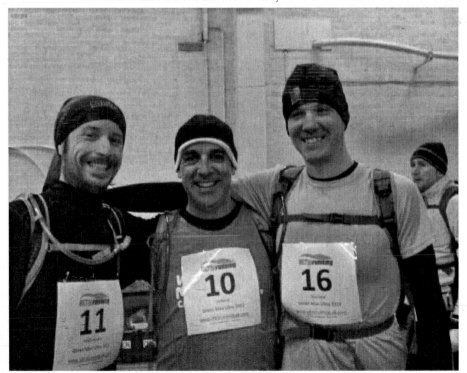

Bear, me and Guy still looking keen and fresh at the start of the Green Man Ultra.

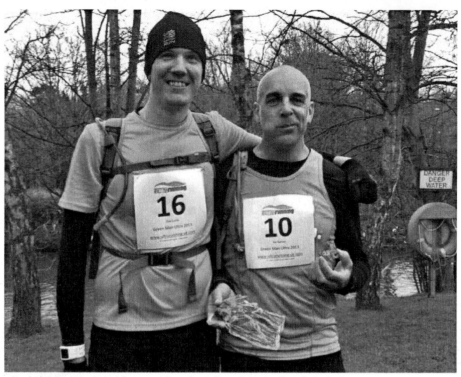

Guy and me munching down fruitcake at the Keynsham checkpoint.

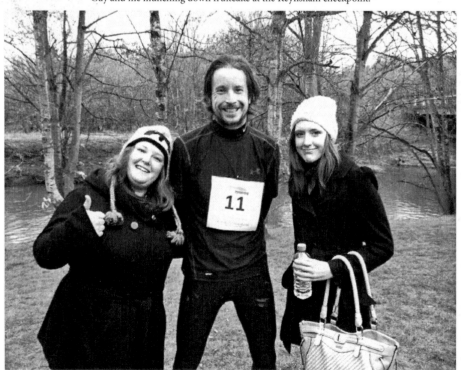

Fay, Bear and Helen at checkpoint two in Keynsham.

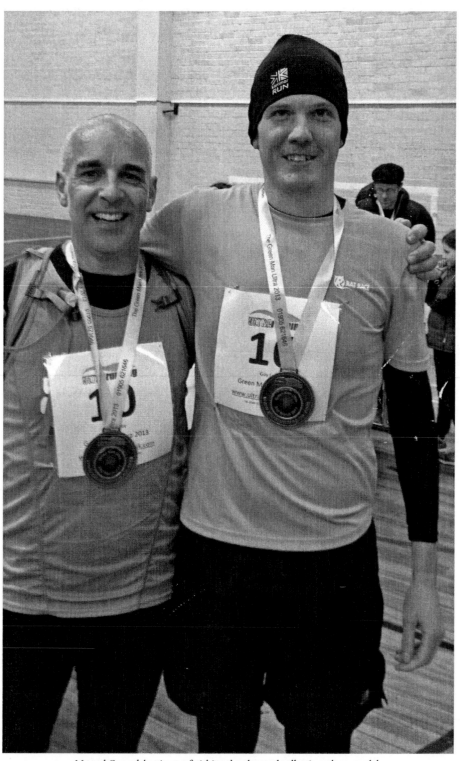

Me and Guy celebrating on finishing the ultra and collecting a huge medal.

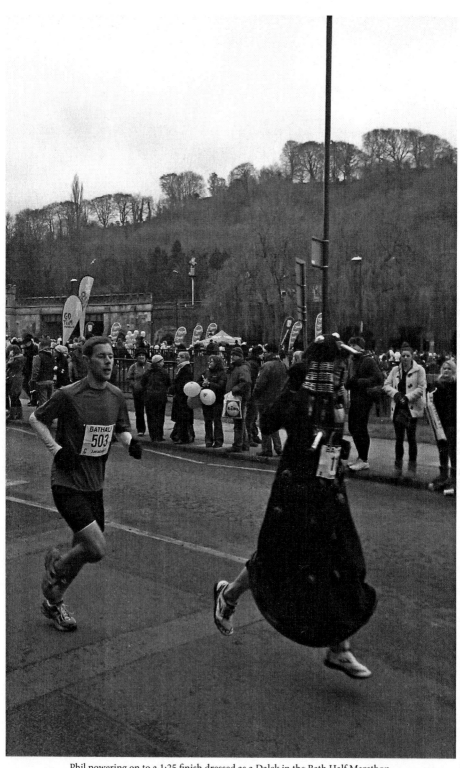

Phil powering on to a 1:25 finish dressed as a Dalek in the Bath Half Marathon.

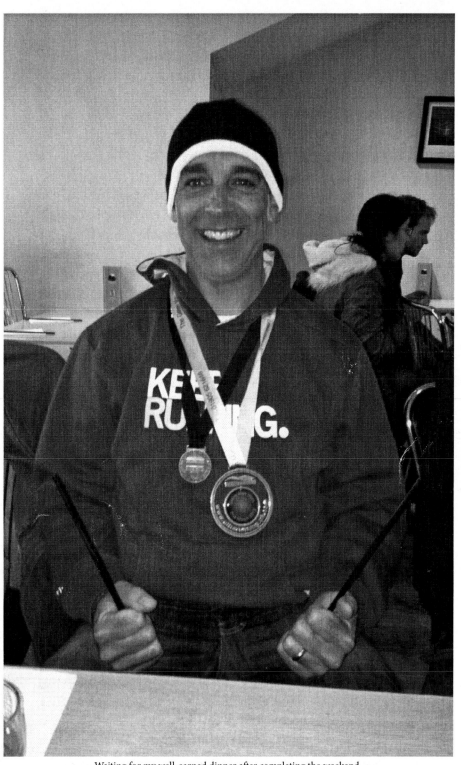

Waiting for my well-earned dinner after completing the weekend.

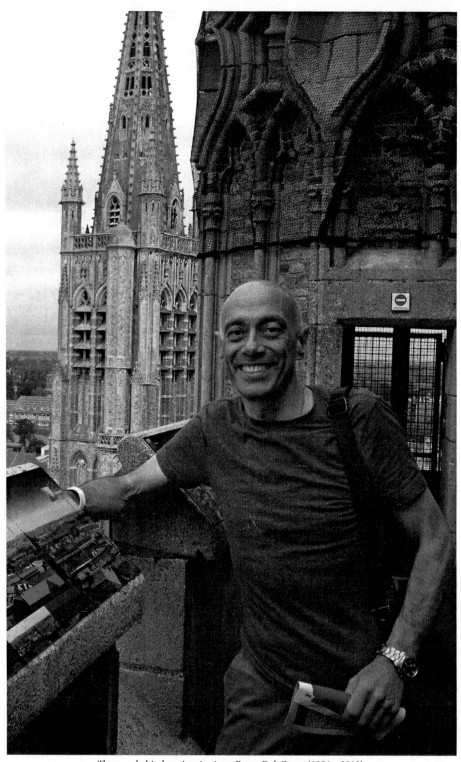

The man behind my inspiration - Remo Del-Greco (1954 – 2013).

to lack motivation some days and whenever I felt like that I would push myself to run through it and often felt better for it afterwards. Other days nothing can get you out of the mire.

Arriving at Warmley Station to meet up with Andy I instantly noticed how it felt really cold for the first time. The dashboard in my car told me it was -1 degrees and stepping out of the car there was no reason to doubt it was working just fine. By the start of the month my weight had fallen to 14st 7lb, meaning I had lost nearly two stone, making a huge difference to my running. I was slowly becoming less of a fat man with each passing day which perhaps unsurprisingly also had the side effect of me really starting to feel the cold more. As usual when running in winter I had kitted myself out appropriately, layering a long-sleeved thermal base layer, long-sleeved top, jacket, tights, fleece hat and gloves. At first that seemed fine but as we got further into the run, moving out into the countryside the temperature dropped noticeably, turning bitterly cold. Despite running a steady pace and being well wrapped up I was finding it difficult to keep myself warm. Other than being bloody cold, the run itself was pretty uneventful. We plodded and chatted our way around the route until we rolled back into Warmley and after saying goodbye I jumped back into my car and cranked the heaters right up. Even with the inside of the car quickly starting to feel like the Sahara however I still felt cold. By the time I had driven the two miles home I started to feel decidedly unwell and was shivering badly. My core felt cold and no amount of layers seemed to make a difference. I stuck a digital thermometer in my ear to be told my temperature was only 35.1 degrees – a good 1.5 degrees below what I should have been. A temperature of 35 degrees or less is classified as hypothermia. I felt awful. I decided to wrap myself up in a thermal base layer, hooded-top, hat and fleecy dressing gown and lie on the sofa for the best part of the rest of the day, sleeping, drinking tea and generally trying to warm up. By late afternoon my temperature had risen to 35.5 degrees and by evening it had climbed back to 36.1 degrees. I was starting to feel better although had lost the best part of a day. What struck me was that although it hadn't been that cold out – I had ran on days much colder than that – a combination of the temperature and a distinct thinning of my insulating body fat over the previous couple of months had seen me start to notice the cold like I had never done before. There was also a likelihood I hadn't eaten enough before the run. Eating itself has a thermogenic effect, in that the process of digestion alone generates heat, which can be important on a cold day to help keep your core temperature up. Add to that the fact that my body would also then have fewer calories readily to hand to work with and you can see how skipping breakfast could have contributed to the problem. Whilst being lighter was enabling me to run faster and train harder, I made a mental note to be more careful over the colder months to make sure this didn't happen again. If there is one thing to be said for being fat, it's that you don't ever feel that cold in the winter.

The end of November and start of December had seen a few really quiet weeks in terms of miles for a number of reasons. The cold weather had bitten hard into the training, plus my wife's shifts also clashed with my planned schedule which couldn't be helped. It's just something that happens when you have to balance family life with a lot of training. For some reason I had also started to feel a touch melancholic which put me into a general mood of apathy towards a lot of things, particularly running. I looked up and read a few articles suggesting that weight loss can affect your mood, for a wide range of reasons. Maybe that was it. I didn't honestly know whether it was the weight loss, the cold weather, or even a touch of overtraining that was causing it. Part of me thought it could be something to do with Remo as some five months in from his initial diagnosis, his health appeared to be deteriorating more quickly now. Whenever I saw him he looked a shadow of the man he was. It was

and for as illuminating as our headtorches were the field was a dark abyss. Having already run the route a few times we knew the general direction we needed to be heading in and squelched our way up towards the stile leading out of the field. The ground was boggy at best and trying to run uphill proved a real challenge. So much so we ended up walking. As we climbed the stile and started to plod our way up the rocky tree-covered gully towards North Stoke, it dawned on me how bonkers this all was. Here we were, two guys simply on our way to the office, commuting by running uphill through a dark wood, shin-deep in mud, in the pouring rain. It was pure horror film stuff. All I needed was to look back and see that Bear had silently vanished, or even worse had pulled a blood-stained axe from his backpack and had a crazed look in his eye. I decided not to look back and just kept plodding upwards, calling back occasionally to make sure he was still there. With the sun not rising until after eight it was still dark, windy and raining as we made our way along the rest of the footpath and down into Bath. Overall the run might have been hard going in places and yes by the time we got to work we were cold, extremely wet and muddy and pretty tired, but it was definitely good Green Man training. In a twisted way it was also strangely satisfying and helped to start shifting my mood back in the right direction.

Despite the end of the year looming we had still run only one short section of the actual Green Man route, so the following weekend I arranged with Bill for Bear and I to run with him to recce a big section of the path, from Pensford through to Keynsham. However, after making plans on where to all meet Bill was forced to pull the plug at the last-minute as the weather had been so wet. As it turned out a large part of the route we had planned to run followed the River Chew but with all the rain almost the entire stretch of footpath was deep under water. The bad weather was really starting to hamper getting out and learning the route. Even when it wasn't raining the ground was so wet from when it had been it was too soft to run on. It was very far from ideal. The year so far had been exceptionally wet and the winter looked set to continue that trend with flood warnings in place all over the UK. Much of the South West remained on alert over Christmas. It was incredible, we started the year with the driest period for one-hundred years, but now it had turned officially into the wettest year on record. All we could do was hope it was going to improve, or our knowledge of the path was going to be poor at best. At worst the event itself could even be at risk.

After the run with Bill was canned Bear and I decided to get out and run the last section of the route from Blaise Castle to Ashton Court, especially seeing as how a large part of it looked as if it was on road and was on pretty high ground, so shouldn't be too wet. How wrong we were.

Saturday morning I got up early, and not having a proper map holder to waterproof my OS map I decided to fold it onto the relevant section and wrap it in Clingfilm. We'd spent the previous afternoon studying the short section of route online and had memorised a bit about how it looked from a bird's eye view. So armed with a map wrapped like a sandwich and our dubious digital memories we were ready. I drove to Bear's house on the other side of Bristol to collect him, before driving on to Blaise Castle. As we pulled up in the car park we sat there for a few minutes watching the rain attacking the ground with full force. All of a sudden the idea of running eight miles seemed ridiculous. Unperturbed, we got out of the car and headed off towards the woods in search of a footpath. This was our first mistake. Whilst we were going generally in the right direction, we entered the woods at the wrong point. This simple mistake meant that we ran about a mile and a half through the woods on the wrong footpath before realising we weren't going the right way. Realising we must have taken the wrong path; we climbed up between the trees eventually finding the clearing we were looking for. Having only covered a couple of miles or so, and already being completely sodden through, we decided it would be a good idea to head back through the woods to see if we could find the start of the path. Wrong again. We couldn't find the right start to the path but having found the clearing we needed we ran back up to it and carried on right down the middle until we came to the iron bridge crossing the road. We crossed the bridge and picked back up on the Community Forest Path signs turning left and following the signs down through Shirehampton Park Golf Club. Yet again I found myself running across a golf course on a Saturday morning plastered in mud. It was becoming a habit. Leaving the golfers behind we crossed the road and straight into a grubby section of footpath that ran behind a series of houses. Clearly the residents didn't realise (or care) it was a public footpath and treated it like a dump. The path was strewn with rubbish: bits of vacuum cleaners, broken toys, even an old pram. It was pretty shabby and far from one of the highlights of Bristol's distributed woodland. Running on through we came out in Sea Mills where we followed more footpath signs up towards Sneyd Park and eventually over Durdham Downs. Being one of the most affluent areas of Bristol it was a world away from the dumping ground we had run through only a couple of miles earlier. By this time it was raining pretty hard but nearing the finish we ran on regardless, following the road down to probably Bristol's best known landmark, the Clifton Suspension Bridge. In all of my years living in Bristol I had never actually walked or run across the bridge. Despite the fact that it was an extremely wet and murky day, running over it was uplifting, partly because of the outstanding view and partly because it meant we were almost done. Over the bridge we entered the Ashton Court Estate and ran into the red deer enclosure, stumbling across the Green Man head. This was it, this was where the name of the race originated. Despite throwing it down with rain, we

running was both appalling and hugely attractive at the same time. After being cooped up indoors for two days straight I felt like I was starting to go stir crazy. I had read three books about ultrarunning in as many days, which was only making me more itchy to get out the door irrespective of the weather. It was late afternoon by the time I stepped out and kicking off up the road it felt great to be running. My legs felt light, as if I hadn't run in weeks, although it had only in fact been four days. Whether it was the release of actually getting out the house or being able to run after reading so much about running over the previous few days, I loved it. I ran six miles around the wet and windswept streets at a good average pace before heading back home to dry off with my mood lifted.

As the year was coming to an end, I found my general disposition was improving. It had been a diabolical month for training if you were counting miles, but the off-road nature of many of the runs had really laid a solid foundation for what was to come in a mere two months. There was still much work to be done before I would be able to take on the challenge but moving into 2013 I was feeling pretty positive about the whole thing. I was certainly going to be starting the year in good running form, quite how good I was about to find out.

11. Unfinished Business

"The best pace is suicide pace, and today looks like a good day to die."
– **Steve Prefontaine**

Sitting at the dinner table in my mother-in-law's house I straighten myself up and exhale slowly in a desperate bid to try and create extra space for the second helping of dinner I'd just consumed. What seemed like such a great idea when I was asked if I wanted to try the succulent beef as well as the juicy lamb (not to mention the double dessert), was now very clearly not. Experience told me that my self-inflicted bellyache will subside in due time – so long as my stomach didn't explode first – I just needed to sit very still and breath slowly through it. Just don't move.

It was the evening of December 27th 2012 and we were fast approaching the end of the Christmas break as well as the end of yet another year. On the whole I had been much more moderate than I have ever been over the festive period, a changed mindset and impending ultramarathon had largely kept my former gluttony at bay without any significant effort or restraint. Dinner at Gill's however seemed to have been the exception. In itself this excessive feasting wouldn't normally be a problem, sure, give yourself a bit of leeway and let yourself go a little every now and then – stuff your face then go home and sleep it off, but on this particular occasion I was beginning to wonder if I really shouldn't have been a touch more cautious, if only for what was to follow in a matter of mere hours – trying to run the fastest five kilometres I had ever attempted.

It was September 2011 when the disaster struck. When I say disaster, I guess I need to be relative – in the scale of world events it didn't rival a major earthquake or famine but in my own little insular running world with my own personal goals and self-imposed importance it certainly seemed like the end of the world at the time. I was ploughing through the final weeks of a training program in preparation for the upcoming Abingdon Marathon in October. It wasn't the first time I'd raced at Abingdon, I'd previously run the race in 2010, smashing my previous marathon best by some twenty minutes, running the pancake-flat two-lap course in an admirable 3 hours 46 minutes. That first year I had followed a training plan set out for me by Bill Graham and everything had gone just as it should have. I lost a bit of weight, trained well and good conditions on the day meant everything just fell into place. Having previously suffered two horrific London Marathons where I went out much too fast and paid the price later, my first Abingdon was like a dream. It was the first marathon I managed to run all the way, as well as avoiding hitting the dreaded wall. My goal that year – as always – had been to try and scrape under the magical four hour barrier and my training had all been geared towards that. About a week before the race however Bill pulled me to one side and suggested that I should go out faster and try for 3 hours 45 minutes. Initially I laughed in his face at such a ridiculous suggestion, especially given that was the time I had always strived for but failed to achieve in London. Bill seemed convinced, so not being the argumentative type I bowed to his greater experience and nervously pledged to give it my best on the day. A much smaller race than London, Abingdon attracts somewhere in the order of 1000 runners over London's 30,000, which meant not getting caught up in crowds over the first few miles, making running a consistent pace much easier from the off. As it turned out Bill's vision was spot on – I was indeed capable of going faster than I realised. Following his advice I tried to run each

be black and blue, I saw nothing. That was it, I had to face up to the fact that I needed help, professional help – I needed to go and see a doctor.

Like many men I never relish a visit to the doctor. I tended not to go if I could help it at all, largely because when I did they always told me I was overweight and drank too much. I already knew all of that I didn't need somebody else telling me as well. It was my slacker attitude at play again, not taking responsibility for my own health. It was easier to think that it would all be alright and that maybe part of me really was bionic and indestructible, which also conveniently played to my fear of mortality. If I was somehow part man, part machine, I didn't actually have to face up to the issue of death – particularly my own. Luckily I'm not often sick enough to require a trip to the surgery but whenever I did go it almost always scared the living crap out of me.

In 2005 I entered the Paris Half Marathon and a condition of entry was a signed letter from a doctor stating you were fit and well enough to run the race. So I made an appointment at my GP's surgery and popped along expecting to be in and out with an autographed note in hand within a few minutes, however the very efficient Austrian doctor with supersonic hearing I saw had other ideas.

"No, I'm sorry, I cannot authorise you to run this race. You have a heart murmur" he said calmly. Slap! A what? Heart what? No! What? The colour drained from my face and thoughts of death instantly flashed through my mind. I didn't know what a heart murmur was but it sounded bad – it had the word heart in the title. Seeing me turn ashen-faced before him he explained it was nothing to really worry about but I did need to get it checked out further before he could give me any kind of letter. Didn't this man know I was a runner? I ran all the time. I might have been fat but how could I have a heart condition, I was a runner. I slowly walked home from the

surgery and without saying a word the second I walked through the front door my wife knew something was up. My face was still so pale it could have been used for colour matching Dulux brilliant white – gloss if you factored in the cold sweat. A week or so later, still alive and thanks to the miracle of modern medical insurance I had an appointment at The Glen hospital in Bristol to see a cardiologist. She ran me through all kinds of scans and tests and confirmed the diagnosis of the Austrian jury. Yes, I did indeed have a heart murmur although one so minor it wasn't worth worrying about. As she was telling me I would live, my emotions became very mixed. I was over the moon that I wasn't actually going to die at any minute however also slightly saddened to find out that I really wasn't indestructible. Whilst I would go on to run the Paris Half Marathon that year (1 hour 50 minutes), a small piece of my personal delusion died that day.

Back at the surgery, a mere four weeks before Abingdon 2011 – making very sure not to see the same Austrian doctor – I presented my super sore feet for inspection to the consulting GP. The diagnosis was swift and simple – classic plantar fasciitis – an inflammation of the fibrous connective tissue on the sole of the foot. It's a common injury, particularly amongst runners but one that can be surprisingly difficult to treat if not looked after correctly. I was already several weeks down the line of trying to ignore it and it wasn't going anywhere, so I was looking for a quick and magical solution to the problem. Something to keep me running for the next few weeks and through the race – some pills, a stretch maybe, in fact anything that would make it just go away really quickly.

The doctor however seemed to take a different approach: *"The best thing you can do Mr Rainey is to simply rest for a good few weeks, take a course of anti-inflammatories and try to keep both feet elevated whenever you can."* Rest? I can't rest; I'm running a marathon in four weeks. Didn't she hear me tell her that at the start? I'd half-heartedly invested a lot of time in this race, I couldn't quit now. Deciding that she probably did know better than me, I took her treatment advice on-board, but with a race to run I thought I would compromise a little. I would sit with my feet up a little bit more and run just a little bit less than my plan dictated. It was only another few weeks, it would be fine, I could rest as much as I liked after the race.

Race day arrived and having had to pare down my training more than I had hoped over the previous few weeks – a kind of enforced tapering as I liked to think of it – the plantar had actually eased up somewhat. Whilst I knew I wasn't in the shape I should've been, I did feel confident of at least getting round – hopefully in less than four hours. Starting off I kept a steady pace and things seemed to be going well, I was running slower than I had wanted to be but I was happy to be there at all after the threat of not even making it to the start line. Everything was going well right up until I needed to stop to relieve myself around the thirteen mile mark. That was when, standing urinating into a hedge with several other men somewhere in the Oxfordshire countryside, I noticed that both my feet were actually really hurting – quite badly. Bad news, the plantar was back with a vengeance. I put negative thoughts to the back of my head and tried to run on but my feet had stopped working properly. Every step I took felt like some mischievous child had inserted another small piece of Lego into my shoes. I battled with thoughts of stopping, telling myself that I was already over halfway and I just needed to keep going. I ran by a St. Johns Ambulance crew, resisting the urge to stop and climb into the back of the ambulance, past another group of marshals and on through the fifteen mile mark where the course looped back around for the second lap. By this time my pace had slowed dramatically from running nine minute miles to nearly sixteen. The reality of the injury was hitting hard and as I hobbled around a corner close to the sixteen mile mark and saw a marshal standing on the side of the road, I made the heart-

decided to enrol the services of Helen, one of the personal trainers at the gym. Helen Hinsley was somebody who I already knew as she was also a member of Bitton Road Runners. She was a good runner, having won the club championships a number of times over the years and someone who I had myself had a few racing battles with in the past. She was the ideal person to try to help me back to fitness and back to running.

What I hadn't bargained for however was quite how unfit I was. The first training session I had with her started with a weigh-in – 16st 10lbs. Ouch, bad start. Then we followed that up with a general fitness assessment with a short but hard bike interval session, blast on the cross-trainer, bit of rowing, all followed up by a range of simple freestyle floor work. An hour later I was a physical wreck, sweating from places I never knew it was possible to sweat from and aching all over. I thought this was about as bad as it could get. I was close to the heaviest I had ever been, I couldn't run, had bad feet and could barely do two press-ups without my arms giving out – and even they were on my knees. Several weeks passed as we moved into January 2012 and I kept up the program with Helen. Improvements were being made and I was starting to notice a bit of a difference. That's when my hip decided to give up on me. At first it was just a niggle, which quite quickly turned into real pain. Within a matter of a couple of weeks it turned into a limp and before I knew it I could do nothing at all, even walking up and down stairs became painful. Clearly I was wrong before, there was always further to fall, although right now I felt like I was at rock bottom.

Being an optimist, the only way to go from rock bottom is up and that is exactly where I intended to go. The first thing I decided to do was to make an appointment to see physiotherapist Dave Adler. On the first appointment I explained to him about my hip and ran through the whole story from plantar through marathon DNF to gym membership. *"You should've just come to see me when the plantar came on,"* he said, *"I treat plantar every week; it's such a common injury."* Great – a little bit less ignoring problems when they crop up and a little bit more actually doing something about them could have quite possibly averted this whole sorry situation it seemed. After a relatively quick bit of prodding, bending and pushing, an over-tight and weakened glutus medius was diagnosed as the likely root of the problem. Much stretching, rubbing and loosening up followed which whilst bloody painful at the time did start to improve things from the off. Following working on the glutes Dave turned his attention to the plantar starting with some deep tissue massage and ultrasound treatment on both feet to help clear up the hard tissue that had formed through my abuse and neglect of the problem since September. By the time I left I felt more positive about everything. I was still a hobbling wreck, but a hobbling wreck that was on the mend.

Within a few weeks of stretching and visits back to Dave, along with a gentle reintroduction of exercise at the gym things were starting to improve, so much so that I had switched from using the cross-trainer which I hated, to running slowly on the treadmill. The plantar was on its way out and running started to feel plausible again. I slowly increased the distance I was running over a matter of weeks until I could run for five kilometres. It wasn't fast but I was running again and it felt great. Always looking to push myself and set a benchmark I decided to see how fast I could run 5K as a starting point to improve upon. At peak running fitness years before, I had managed to run a 5K race in just a touch under twenty minutes, which I was extremely pleased with at the time. In all the years since I'd never managed to get anywhere close to that and wondered if I ever would. That day in the gym I ran 28 minutes 40 seconds for five kilometres and it nearly killed me. This was to be my benchmark going forward. But if that was where I was, where did I want to be? What was my goal? Never one to shy away from a challenge,

conditions. If I could get into a gym then I could use a treadmill and get somebody else to witness my run. I wasn't a member any longer, letting my membership expire at the end of November as the year contract expired. That's when the bulb lit above my head – Fitness First had a scheme where an existing member could sign in a guest for free on a Friday – that could work. Today was Wednesday so I had time to work it out. I drew up a shortlist of people who I knew were members of Fitness First and crossed them off if I thought they'd be busy at Christmas time. After a few minutes I was left with just two names, Phil and Scott. Knowing that Phil went to the gym most days he was always an option but I wasn't sure if he was away for the festive season, whereas I knew Scott was working on Friday and often went to the gym before work anyway. A quick text conversation and it was arranged. We would meet on Friday 28th December at seven o'clock outside Fitness First in Bath where he would sign me in as a guest and witness my humble effort at destroying myself on a treadmill mere days before the year was over.

As my alarm went off at six o'clock the morning after the all-you-can-eat feeding at Gill's I rolled out of bed still feeling like I wouldn't need to eat for most of that day. I supped on a cup of strong coffee to wake myself up, packed my kit bag and headed off to Bath. On the drive over I questioned myself as to what I thought I might be able to achieve. The delusional optimist in me had faith in my ability to smash the time and walk away victorious but there was also a niggling voice of realism in the back of my head telling me I would be shooting off the back of that treadmill after about five minutes whilst vomiting both succulent beef and juicy lamb over the control panel on my way down. If anybody had a video camera to hand there was a sure £250 in it from You've Been Framed. After signing into the gym, it was pretty clear that unless Scott had a video camera that nobody was making any money today, as the gym was deserted. It was early and still in that pre-New Year binge period before people headed to the gym in their hordes. Quiet was good, less people to see me make a twat of myself. In preparation I ran a single kilometre at a slow pace to warm myself up, went to the bathroom and came back ready for the main event. Scott was on the treadmill next to me and was also going to time me as well as using the timer on the machine itself.

I had worked out that to run under nineteen minutes I would need to run each kilometre at no less than 3 minutes 47 seconds (which equates to 6 minutes 5 seconds per mile). This wouldn't give me any leeway, so perhaps a bit quicker would be a better, if somewhat tougher option. We both decided that because it takes time to build up to a set speed that we should set the treadmill going at 16kph (giving me a possible time of 18 minutes 47 seconds) and let it build right up to speed before jumping onto a moving belt. It sounded like a good idea, but at the same time like a pretty stupid one, this was definitely YBF territory.

So it was with a belt moving at a seemingly ridiculous pace and Scott laughing next to me, I took a deep breath and jumped from the sides onto the belt and ran like I'd stolen something. The initial action of switching from standing still to running six minute miles was indeed a little tricky, however once I got my legs moving at the same speed as the belt I was fine. Challenge one complete, now I just had to keep going. After my body got over the initial shock of what I was asking of it I settled down into a rhythm, breathing steadily and trying to keep my legs moving whilst distracting my mind from what I was trying to do. There was no Jeremy Kyle on the TV this early but a range of senseless music videos provided some relief while my lungs tried desperately to catch up with my legs. I was a good two kilometres down before it started to get tough, but bearing it out until two and a half I knew I was over halfway and I had less left to do than I had already done. This was going well – almost too well. It certainly wasn't easy but as I smashed my way through the third kilometre I could see the end, I just needed to keep it going and get it over with now. I was sweating profusely, my breathing was shallow and my legs were starting to flag, which is why I made the executive decision as I hit the 4K mark to push the speed up. It might have seemed counter-intuitive however my thinking was the faster I ran the faster this would be over. I had less than one kilometre to go as I pushed the speed up to 16.5kph and then again up to 17.5kph. I figured it was go for broke time. As my legs span like Scooby Doo escaping a baddie I watched the odometer slowly climb its way up to the required five kilometres. As soon as the big hand pointed to five I smashed the stop button and immediately jumped to the sides, trying to stay upright and not empty my still full stomach over the slowing belt. Scott checked his watch – 18 minutes 29 seconds. Boom! I had done it and with time to spare. Once I managed to catch my breath, I was slightly taken aback at just how fast I'd run – 3.1 miles at an average pace of 5 minutes 56 seconds per mile. That was by far and away the fastest I had ever run anything, and whilst I knew that running on a treadmill was a little bit easier than out in the real world, it was vindication enough for me of achieving my goal for 2012. It was a great way to end the year and proved – just as Bill suggested I did back in Abingdon – that sometimes you need to take a chance and push yourself beyond what you think you are capable of to really find out what you can achieve.

12. Training Diary: January

"Ask yourself: 'Can I give more?'. The answer is usually: 'Yes'."
– **Paul Tergat**

Total Miles Run: 137.50
Highest Weekly Total: 39.00
Weekly Average: 31.04

As we moved into the New Year I became acutely aware of the fact that we were now only a mere two months away from the Green Man and although weight loss and training had been going well, we had only managed to run two short sections of the route. Perhaps unsurprisingly I had also gained a few pounds over Christmas, which would require more effort to lose and to cap things off, my mileage tally for December was absolutely shocking. I really needed to start ramping up the long miles. So far the longest I had run in training was fifteen miles, which whilst not an insignificant distance, it was such a very long way from forty-six. I decided to rectify this and start the year off with a symbolic gesture of mileage, by jumping straight up to running twenty miles on New Year's Day. I had run this far a number of times when training for a marathon but hadn't been anywhere close to it for at least eighteen months. With it being New Year, candidates ready and willing to run a stupid amount of miles on a bank holiday were somewhat thin on the ground, with so many of them having drank and partied the night away until the early hours. The two people I knew who wouldn't have been drinking were Bear and Phil. Simply because Bear doesn't drink and Phil couldn't drink due to various medication. However Bear was away, which left me with just Phil as an option. Luckily, when it came to running a long way, Phil was generally a pretty good option, having accompanied me on most of my twenty mile runs in the past. As it turned out, this one was going to be no different.

I first met Phil Westlake when we started working together in 1999. At that time I hadn't even started running but Phil was already a force to be reckoned with. A familiar story, he started running, aged twenty-three, after deciding to lose weight and run a half marathon. During his first training run he had to stop on an old couple's garden wall, trying hard not to vomit into their carefully tended flower bed. After a brief chat with the concerned pensioners he turned around and walked the mile back home, deflated. Never one to give up, he persevered with training and finished his first half marathon in a very respectable 1 hour 30 minutes. Some years later, after a family-induced hiatus, he joined Bitton Road Runners, where his indefatigable competitiveness drove him to train incessantly, setting him on course to win the club championship several times as well as setting new senior male club records in six out of the eight recorded distances. His 'flat out from the start' approach to running worked well over shorter distances but over longer runs his self-admitted lack of pace judgement always hampered his best times – not that that stopped him trying anyway. After a number of years running near the front of the pack, he took a break from competitive running in 2004, continuing running merely to keep fit and it was largely during this time that we would go out on long Sunday morning runs. Regardless of what I was training for, or how far or fast I wanted to run, Phil was always there willing to pace me, keeping me going through the tough miles. Quite simply I wouldn't be the runner I am today without his help over the years and I will always be grateful to him for that.

troponin level was abnormally high and suspected he had suffered a heart attack. Doctors concluded this was almost certainly down to his heart having reverted into AF and continuing to stress it by his insistence to complete the race. It wasn't great news, which resulted in a second cardioversion and a new course of anti-coagulants and beta-blockers, this time however for much longer, possibly for life. Of all the drugs for a runner to be put on, beta-blockers are far from ideal. In essence they prevent the heart working at its maximum, restricting blood flow to muscles that need it. As a result, running is much harder work and it essentially caps your performance. Essentially, this brought Phil's competitive running career to an end. But as was the way when he had stepped out of racing in 2004, he continued to maintain a fairly high training mileage, albeit now largely indoors. As before however, when I needed somebody to help drag my lazy fat ass around more miles than I was ready for, Treadmill Phil – as he was now better known – was there to help.

After such shocking weather in December, it was sheer joy to get out and run on such a dry clear day as it was on New Year's day. It was as if the sun had quite literally woken for the start of the year. Whilst the morning was bathed in sunshine it was far from warm, setting off at eight o'clock it was still cold and after my suffering the previous month I made sure to wrap up well – intent on not spending another afternoon lying on the sofa feeling like crap. Mildly trepidatious about the distance I was about to undertake, I loaded my backpack up with water; cereal bars; mini-cheddars; and a handful of digestive biscuits to munch on along the way and set out to meet Phil. We ran a slow steady loop from Kingswood, down through Bitton, Wick, Pucklechurch, Shortwood, through Warmley and back up to Kingswood, with a couple of stops along the way to fuel up on my savoury stash and stretch my hips which had started to tighten up after about five miles. We paced it steadily, running around a nine minute mile average and I was surprised how far we got before I

me, with Jon sprinting out twenty seconds behind her. By the time I started running I had already lost sight of the others along the twists in the river path. Wearing my Garmin I knew how far along the path I had gone, but I had also marked out on a map the quarter-mile points, so I could easily break the distance down into roughly four-hundred metre chunks as I was running. Sprinting off from the start line it felt great to be running fast. It is satisfying finishing a long run but there really is nothing quite like the feeling of shifting along at breakneck speed under your own steam. Half a mile in and the smiles and joy rapidly faded as my body realised what my head was trying to get it to do. Running around a six minute mile pace, it wasn't until I saw the green bridge at the mile turning point come into view that I saw Rebecca and Jon ahead of me. They were both running hard and still held a good lead on me however being the closest to me they were my targets for today and I was determined to reel them in. Slapping my hand on the bridge and turning I clocked six minutes and fifteen seconds for the first mile and bounded off after everyone already well on their way back to the finish line. Really blowing, I tried hard to keep the speed up and as I went through a mile and a half I pushed on harder figuring it was now or never. I was tired but I figured so must everybody else be. According to the GPS I was still running just over six minute mile pace as I finally caught Jon with just over a quarter mile to go. I slowly edged by him and strode on in a desperate attempt to catch Rebecca who was really moving. With less than fifty metres to go and the finish line closing fast I just managed to dip in front of her, finishing the second mile in six minutes and nine seconds, giving me a time of twelve minutes and twenty four seconds for the two miles. I was pleased. I was shattered and lying on the tarmac with my lungs burning but I was pleased. I had never run that fast outside before and it was a sure sign of big improvements in my fitness. Everyone who took part posted better than expected times, pushing themselves hard not to be caught. Could they all sustain it going forward?

The following week, despite running most days, I only managed to clock up around twenty-five miles. Part of that mileage though did include a second, better-attended handicap challenge, with around a dozen people making the effort to push themselves and running more great times, all being pretty consistent with the first week. It was working well and getting people running faster.

With the weather improving slightly Bear and I decided to jump in with both feet and have another crack at recceing an unfamiliar fifteen mile section of the Green Man route – from Ashton Court Estate, near the start of the race, to the Lock Keeper pub in Keynsham, where the second checkpoint would be on race day. Whilst we had run further on the road, this was the real deal. Not only was it the actual Green Man route but it was on the real terrain too, which given all the rain we had suffered recently, was pretty boggy underfoot.

I always think running point-to-point is mentally easier than going out on a loop, as you can't simply dip out and cut off a corner to shorten your run when you don't feel like doing it all. However you feel, you still have to get from A to B. While this might be physically demanding if you're not in the mood, mentally you know you don't have a choice so you just get on with it. The trouble with this section of the route though was that it wasn't really close to either of our houses, so required a touch of logistical planning. We decided to meet at Keynsham, where we would leave one car behind before driving over to Ashton Court on the other side of Bristol to start the run. On finishing we would then drive back from Keynsham in the car we had left behind, back to Ashton Court to collect the other car before driving home again. It wasn't convoluted at all. So, at seven o'clock on a cold dark Sunday morning I rolled up at the Lock Keeper in Keynsham to meet Bear. Not only Bear though – today we would also be joined by another ultramarathon novice and

Green Man challenger, Guy Lucas.

Guy was a friend of Scott's from Frome, who had only been running a couple of years. Impossibly tall and generally fit, he had originally been inspired to get into shape and try his hand at running after watching Eddie Izzard run forty-three marathons in fifty-one days. He started slow, building up his mileage with a pipe dream of one day managing to run a 10K. As with most people who get bitten by the running bug however, that goal pretty quickly came and went, seeing him pass complete a half marathon, a twenty-mile road race and an off-road marathon before being talked into running the Green Man by Bear – and all within the space of two years. Now he found himself in the car park of a pub, in a small market town between Bristol and Bath, early on a chilly Sunday morning in January and planning on spending the best part of the next three hours running through muddy fields back to this very spot. Welcome to Green Man training.

For the first time we had decided to use the official race directions which on the face of it looked pretty verbose. This quickly proved to be their redeeming feature though as the detail was exactly what was needed to find our way. Setting off from Ashton Court around twenty past eight, the sun was coming up and the grass was frosty white and crispy underfoot as we followed the Community Forest Path out of the estate, down towards the A370 and Dundry Hill. It was one of those clichéd moments when you paused to think: this is why I run. It was dawn, there was a wintery chill in the air and we were still fresh and keen for adventure. It doesn't get any better than this. Remembering moments like that are what keep you going through the tough miles. Romantic dreaming over, it only took a couple of miles for the route to turn seriously wet and boggy and the pleasant chill to morph into just being bloody cold. Before we knew it we were already plastered in mud up to the shin and pretty wet through. We crossed the A38 and attempted to run our way through a rough field that had clearly seen a lot of recent horse and tractor action. Without many footpath signs to follow we waded through the mud, pretending to run, until we found the way out we were looking for, which was a mixed blessing as it also signalled the start of the climb to Dundry – which at around seven-hundred and twenty-two feet is easily the highest point on the route, particularly rising up as it does from almost sea level. Remembering Bill's sage advice on hills we walked the climb, trying to keep the pace steady, but also trying to breathe and chew on a Snickers bar at the same time. Not as easy as it sounds. The reward from the top of the hill (other than flat ground) is an outstanding view that looks out over most of south and central Bristol. From up there you can appreciate how big a city it is – and here we were planning on running all the way around it.

Leaving Dundry village, we met up with Jon who planned to run with us through to Pensford and consulting the laminated sheet of A4 instructions carefully we found our way down through a myriad of unfamiliar country lanes, farms and fields, stopping briefly en-route to scoff on an assortment of energy-filled goodies. Still trying out fuel ideas to see what worked we polished off an assortment of banana sandwiches, energy bars and oatmeal and peanut butter balls between us before setting off again through yet more mud, streams, flooded fields and villages. According to the instructions we ran over an airfield just after checkpoint one at Norton Malreward, which wasn't exactly what I was expecting from the description – it certainly wasn't Heathrow. Still, playing safe we looked both ways (as well as up) before running across the runway and down a rock-strewn gully, across yet another flooded field taking us into the village of Pensford with its familiar omnipresent viaduct. Trying to avoid a huge bull in a small field in the village of Woollard we got lost in a copse of trees before managing to skip around the route (and the bull) joining back onto it before entering some woodland leading us down into Compton Dando. We continued to follow the mud trail along the River Chew plodding all the way down the (until very recently submerged) riverbank to Keynsham, through the park and back to the pub. Arriving at the Lock Keeper we took a well-deserved seat on the wet gravel. It was bloody luxury. Exhausted, we were finally back at the car we had abandoned hours earlier. Having just spent over three hours running little more than fifteen miles of the Green Man route, we were tired, thrilled and a touch overwhelmed. We had managed to successfully recce our biggest section of the course yet but the stark realisation that we had still run less than one third of the total distance of the race brought us back down to Earth with a worrying sense of reality. There were just seven weeks left to learn the rest of the route and to build endurance to the level where we could actually run it all in one go. We had done well but we weren't quite there yet.

One of the few problems of being overly confident is that sometimes, when you are actually wrong, it can come as a something of a shock. On the following Thursday afternoon, I was looking forward to – and planning for – another successful handicap run, with my plan being to run under twelve minutes for the two mile course. However checking the weather forecast, apparently the Met Office had put out a rare red warning for snow the following day. Snow? Pah! It might have been a touch frosty but it certainly wasn't going to snow, it never snows. Nothing to worry about I thought. That was until I got up the following morning and opened the curtains to see my car below five inches of the stuff and it still coming down hard. Bugger. There had been some pre-emptive talk of running a speed session in the gym during lunchtime if the weather was bad but with it being so heavy the schools were all closed and I ended up staying home and looking after the kids. Running would just have to wait, at least for a few days anyway. With so much still to do the idea of wasting days sitting around doing nothing niggled me although there really wasn't anything I could do about it. I tried to convince myself that this could be called a 'rest week' but I wasn't kidding anyone – least of all myself.

Sitting around at home that weekend I thought about Remo and my original reason for undertaking the whole challenge in the first place. A few of us had recently been to see him at home and we sat around chatting for the best part of a couple of hours over lunch and it was great to see him. He was clearly very unwell and looked gaunt. Still his chipper nature persisted and talking to him you would almost never know he was ill. As we left and headed back to work I was pleased to have had the chance to catch up with him, yet saddened to see him slipping away. I was unsure when or even if I would get a chance to see him again.

A week earlier, one of my friends asked me if they could sponsor me for the ultramarathon and I told them I wasn't actually running it for a charity. They said I should, which I considered at the time but promptly forgot. It was as I was sitting around that Sunday evening I realised it would be wrong to not at least try to use this challenge to help raise awareness – and more importantly cold hard cash – for a worthy cancer cause. Remo's diagnosis might have been terminal but anything we could do to help anybody else, however large or small would be worthwhile.

Up until that point the challenge had solely been to run the Green Man, my first ultramarathon, however there had been an ongoing joke that both Bear and Guy were also going to run the Bath Half Marathon the following day. I never considered them as being serious, I mean with so much to tackle on the Saturday, how could they possibly then get up again the following morning and run another thirteen miles? It just wasn't going to happen. But as I sat there, once again, the delusional part of me took over. If they were going to at least try it, then so was I. How hard can it be? We were already pushing the limits of what we were capable of – why not just push it a bit further? Whether or not it was a good idea; whether I would be able to stand up on Sunday; or whether I would just end up limping around the streets of Bath like the Tin Man from the Wizard of Oz, with race marshals camped out in sleeping bags I wasn't sure, but I was sure I was going to give it a try. What had started out as forty-six miles in a loop around Bristol, had just morphed into close to sixty (no I'm not that bad at maths – I was factoring in some leeway), all in a little over a twenty-four hour period.

The following morning I called Macmillan Cancer Support and explained the challenge to them. Always keen to bolster their fundraising team, they happily gave me one of their bond places for the Bath Half Marathon, meaning although the race was long sold out, I was now in. The challenge was on. I setup a donation page at justgiving.com and outlined the weekend and sent it around to a few family and friends, as well as posting a notice about it at work. My target was to attempt to raise £600, making a nice round £10 per mile for the weekend. I don't generally like asking people for money, even for good causes, so I thought this could be a challenge in itself, although after I raised close to £400 within the first twenty-four hours, I realised I might have underestimated people somewhat. What was truly amazing and massively humbling at the same time were all the messages of support I received from people sponsoring me and telling me about the people they know and love who had been tragically affected by cancer. The other thing that struck me was just how much people were in awe of what we were doing. It made me take a step back and question if we had not underestimated it all ourselves. I hope we hadn't as now there was other people's money riding on it too.

A few days later, once the snow had largely cleared and we got back to some semblance of training, we resumed our handicap challenge the following Friday. Feeling a bit lethargic at the start after almost a week without training I went out listening to some fast music in a desperate bid to try and conquer my apathy. Whether it was the enforced rest or the tunes that helped I'm not sure but as I hit the bridge and turned around my first mile in five minutes and forty-three seconds, I knew I was either a) going to be on for a good time, or b) going to need to be fished out of the river somewhere along the way back. Chasing Scott and Jon back to the finish I just managed to edge past Jon but never quite caught Scott before the line. I ran eleven minutes and fifty-nine seconds for the two miles, which I was chuffed to bits with, especially seeing as I felt so lethargic at the start. Maybe the enforced week of rest did me some good after all.

On a roll from the successful recce a couple of weeks earlier, the following Sunday we set out to cover a twenty-three mile section from Keynsham to Blaise Estate. The snow was now long gone, leaving in its place yet more mud to contend with but that was going to turn out to be the least of our worries.

With long miles to come, we needed an early start so getting up at six o'clock, I knocked back a bowl of porridge and stepping out of my front door into the dark morning, with rain beating down against the front of the house and the wind howling around it, I wondered what the hell I was doing. After picking up Bear and leaving his car at Blaise, we drove back to Keynsham to meet up with Guy and another Bitton Road Running buddy of mine, Kev Mowat. Over only a short number of years Kev had gone from non-runner to ultrarunner, running marathons and ultras all over the world, even completing the Namib Desert Challenge – a one-hundred and thirty-six mile jaunt over five days in temperatures of up to forty-six degrees. He took a very relaxed view on the whole thing, confirming what I had been told by many people all the way along – that ultrarunning wasn't about racing, it was about seeing how far you can push yourself and experiencing more from your run. Kev's exact words that made me smile were: *"Some silly bugger's organised these races for people like me, running local races all the time seemed small time considering what was out there, stunning locations, great experiences and great people. But more than anything is that feeling when you cross that line."* You just can't argue with that.

With the rain abating and the sun coming up, we set out from the Lock Keeper plodding our way through muddy fields that had up until only a few days before been underwater. We followed the path through Willsbridge Mill and up onto a short section of the Bristol to Bath cycletrack, before taking an old coal dramway path to Warmley, where we met up with the start of the section I had first ran back in November. Being familiar territory we steadily ran the next six miles right through to Winterbourne with using any directions at all, which was surprisingly liberating. As soon as we got past that point however it all went a tad pear-shaped. Taking a steep path down through the woods towards the River Frome we were confronted not as we expected by a pleasant meandering tributary but a murky brown torrent of a river that had totally engulfed the footpath. It had in fact swallowed the whole riverbank, enveloping it like the Lost City of Atlantis. We stood and contemplated a while wondering if we should turn around and find a safer way route or whether to stay true to the path and just keep going. Possibly foolishly we decided to wade on through the newly-widened river with the thinking being that if we stuck close to the fence then we should still be walking where the bank once stood as opposed to in the middle of the river. Should being the key word here, given none of us had ever seen the bank and had no idea how wide or shallow it was. It was all a bit of a laugh at first but as we cautiously edged forward and the water rose up around our waists, all joking temporarily subsided until we found ourselves safely back on dry land. When I say dry, I obviously mean muddy, just not underwater. Smug at having survived being washed away, we pushed on to

Hambrook, the location of checkpoint three on race day and headed off through Stoke Gifford and Bradley Stoke. By this point we had covered close to seventeen miles and we were beginning to flag somewhat. We stopped to refuel on a diet of gels, energy bars and Powerade (taking the science approach for the day) and sat working out how much further we had to go. Then, realising there were still a lot more miles left than we wanted to think about, we simply stopped counting and started running again. I had heard from Bill some weeks before that the footbridge across the M5 motorway at Patchway was being replaced, meaning a long diversion for anyone wanting to stay faithful to the route. Putting a positive spin on it, in my head I naturally assumed that it would be fine by now and even as we ran past big red signs telling us the footpath ahead was closed, I figured somebody had simply forgotten to take them down. A few hundred metres on however and it was clear they hadn't. Whilst the new bridge was indeed in-situ over the motorway, it was still closed off with a metal fence and very clear signage indicating politely that we really should be looking for another way to cross the motorway. Looking at the suggested alternative on the map however we decided that it was just too much to tack onto an already ridiculously long run and maybe we would just take a quick look to see how many people were milling around the bridge building site. As it turned out, there was nobody: no builders; no security; nobody. Needless to say we did make our way to Easter Compton that morning, but under no circumstances did we break into a building site, scale a six-foot fence, run across an unfinished bridge spanning a motorway, before climbing a second fence the other side and run off giggling. We absolutely did not do that, because that would be potentially dangerous, irresponsible and quite possibly even illegal.

The section from Easter Compton to Blaise is probably the toughest and most miserable chunk of the whole route, with most of it being rough muddy woodland, taking you to one of the steepest

13. Training Diary: February

"Don't let fatigue make a coward of you." – **Steve Prefontaine**

Total Miles Run: 109.50
Highest Weekly Total: 34.00
Weekly Average: 27.37

With the worst of the winter weather hopefully behind us we started February with a positive air. It really felt like it was all starting to come together. My weight had still been slowly falling and although it seemed to have plateaued somewhat, I was now down to 13st 12lb –the lightest I had been for as long as I could remember. This had the benefit of not only making running much easier but also allowing a whole different bunch of clothes to fit better. I now had a whole new wardrobe, most of which I had always owned although never actually had been able to wear.

As far as the Green Man was concerned we now knew the route (or at least we thought we did) and although we hadn't been running ridiculous amounts of miles, we had been slowly and successfully building our endurance over the weeks. Our longest run to date had been from Keynsham to Blaise, which came in at around twenty-three miles but we were about to smash that by some distance by spending the first weekend of February with a mammoth back-to-back training session.

All ultrarunning advice I had been given or read said that, if possible, you should attempt to break down the event distance over the span of a couple of consecutive days. The theory of the back-to-back run was to teach you to keep going when you were still tired; allow for at least some recovery; and reduce the risk of injury when covering huge distances. It should also be stated that unless you are very single and have nothing else going on in your life, then running for two days straight is pretty disruptive to normal life, particularly if you have a family. It will blow anything else you might need to do that weekend out of the water. Forget shopping, laundry, or spending any time with your kids, you're going to be running, eating and sleeping for two days straight. That is more or less it. Even when you do finally end up back at home, you'll be fit for nothing. Accept all of that, get your other half to accept it too and you'll probably be just fine.

Saturday morning came around and with cars strategically dumped across Bristol and the sun rising over the Ashton Court Mansion House, Guy, Bear, Kev, myself, together with yet another Bitton Road Runner, Lynette Porter stood in the car park discussing our plans. Despite standing tall in the low five foot something range, Lynette was a very strong and capable runner, who had set a number of fast veteran club records over the years. With performances such as running just over three hours for a road marathon she would normally leave me for dust on a run, but deep mud and short legs are great levellers, the combination of which I hoped would slow her down enough to give the rest of us a chance of survival.

We opted to use the race checkpoints to break down the route for the weekend, planning to run from Ashton Court to the White Horse pub in Hambrook on Saturday, before wearily returning back to Hambrook on Sunday morning and making our way back once again to Ashton Court. This would mean us covering around twenty-seven miles on day one and a slightly softer seventeen for day two (yes I know that doesn't quite add up to forty-six, but

starting to stiffen up somewhat. The continual soft mud was hard going underfoot, giving you nothing back for all the energy it took out of you, which made joining the cycletrack at Bitton pure luxury. The section of the path from Warmley through to Winterbourne was now so recognizable, having already run it four times it passed by like a familiar car journey – without really noticing we had even been there. Even running across the green at the Kendleshire Golf Club didn't raise an eyebrow from anyone. Crossing the main road we followed the path back down to the River Frome, where we had gone paddling the previous month. We were all ready to wade through the waist deep waters once more, carrying Lynette on our shoulders if need be, when we were presented with not a fast flowing torrent as before but a much more sedate scene complete with riverbank – footpath and all. The river was a good metre lower than it had been the last time we were here, which was great news for the race, as it had started to look like it could be under threat with the weather as it had been. With the end now so tantalisingly close, it was only a short tired few miles down a handful of non-descript country lanes between us and the checkpoint at Hambrook and more importantly the end of day one of our weekend. We eventually plodded into the pub car park about ten minutes up on our initial plan, having covered twenty-seven miles in just over five and a half hours. We were ultrarunners. We had just run further than a marathon – merely as a training run – and tomorrow we were going to do close to the same again. It was the kind of thing you read about in books. The kind of thing Karnazes did. It was the furthest distance any of us (with the exception of Kev) had ever run and somehow we were all still in one piece and able to joke about it. As we stood around drinking coffee from a flask and eating leftover Christmas cake that Kev's wife had amazingly turned up with, we laughed at the absurdity of the whole thing. If we had stopped to think about it more I'm sure we would have realised it was something of a big deal but we were all too busy worrying about the next day to pat ourselves on the back at that point in time.

Parting company with the others, for a few hours at least, I drove home to sit in a bath of ice. Despite not being entirely convinced by the idea I had read that ice baths can help aid the recovery of damaged muscle fibres and to be honest anything that could make the next day's running any easier had to be worth a try. I had already run further than I had ever run before and yet I was still planning on getting up early again the next day and running, again further than I normally would. If sitting around in a bit of cold water would help with that then bring it on.

Not really knowing what I was doing and with the internet at my disposal I did a quick search on *"how long should I sit in an ice bath?"* The general consensus seemed to be about ten minutes, so I duly filled the bath with icy cold water deep enough to cover my legs and jumped straight in. Yeeeooooowwww! Pleasant certainly wasn't a word you could use to describe it. I thought for a second that my legs might actually solidify and snap off, but as per the instructions, after I'd been sat there a few minutes and had acclimatised to the temperature, I added the ice and started the timer. I can generally find something to say for most situations but words fail me on the level of discomfort that ice on the rocks delivers, bordering on torture even. All I can remember thinking was that this had better bloody be worth it.

After I managed to climb out of the bath the first thing I noticed (other than blissful warmth), was that during the day I had developed a very sizable patch of undercarriage and two veg chaffing, which I felt most when I got in the shower and doused myself in shower gel. I almost hit the roof with the pain. Twice in one day – this was turning out to be a somewhat masochistic day. After getting out of the shower I liberally applied an industrial coating of Savlon and waded my way to the shops looking like John Wayne and bought a supersize tub of Vaseline ready for the next day's onslaught.

After not sleeping half as much as I would have liked, Sunday morning came around pretty quickly and before I knew it I found myself standing in the kitchen trying to wake myself up with a mixture of coffee, Weetabix and Lucozade Sport. I noticed that I had developed a sizable blister on the inside of my right foot so decided to wrap a chunk of my foot in silver duct tape (something I had read on a website somewhere about ultrarunning), which actually seemed to do the trick of protecting it pretty well. I decided against shielding my man tackle in the same way, sticking with the Vaseline for that. I also noticed that my left ankle felt a little tender, almost as if I had sprained it, which was a bit of a concern. I rotated it around a little and did a few stretches in a desperate bid to try and make the discomfort go away but all to no avail. Ever the hoper I thought I'd try running on it anyway. I'd just take it steady. What harm could there be in that?

Back at Hambook a group of familiar, weary and apprehensive runners gathered ready for round two. Setting off to the sounds of assorted groaning, we were soon hobbling off in the general direction of Bradley Stoke. Today was new ground for all of us and nobody quite knew how the day was going to pan out, but once we got moving our bodies started to loosen up and after a couple of miles it was almost as if we hadn't run the day before at all. My ankle felt a little sore initially although the more I ran, the more it seemed to ease up and in the end I simply forgot about it.

Running the first handful of miles through the largely featureless estates to the north of the city made for good progress as much of it was on tarmac and firm ground and before we knew it we found ourselves back in Patchway at the motorway crossing that had blocked our way the last time. The new bridge was still unfinished and fenced off; still blocking our way; and still devoid of security staff. Once again, being responsible adults, we absolutely did not climb a security fence into a building site with the aim of running across a closed bridge and we most definitely did not have to lift Lynette over the fence because she couldn't climb it. With a mere four weeks to go until the race, it was starting to look touch and go whether or not the bridge would be open in time. The original deadline for completion had been and gone and clearly the project was running late. Failure to be able to cross the motorway at this point on the day could add a hefty chunk of miles onto the route which to be honest we could all do without.

With a shorter route to cover, there was only one checkpoint stop on Sunday, at Blaise Castle, where we stopped and munched down anything that had sugar in it. From Blaise we knew we only had around seven or eight miles to go and despite having a fair amount of climb in it, a lot of it was on firm ground. The combination of solid ground underfoot and the knowledge it was nearly over put a new found spring in our step that carried us through Sea Mills, across Durdham Downs and over Clifton Suspension Bridge back into Ashton Court Estate. There had been some talk earlier in the day about possibly running all the way up to the Redwood Hotel however unsurprisingly as soon as the car park came into sight, nobody seemed that struck on the idea. With our abandoned cars in our sights we bounded down through the deer enclosure with smiles on our faces knowing that we had done it. Over the space of two days we had run the entire Community Forest Path, without instructions and had survived to tell the tale. We felt pretty pleased with ourselves. Stopping in the car park and sitting on the ground, safe in the knowledge that we didn't have to run again that weekend, we relaxed and revelled in what we had achieved. All of a sudden it felt real and within our grasp. We had completed the back-to-back challenge, covering forty-four miles over both days. On race weekend all we need to do would be the same again – only Saturday would just be a tiny bit longer.

The following morning I woke with legs that felt distinctly like they were owned by somebody else. To top it off the sore ankle was back and if anything a little worse that it was the day before. I thought I would take a couple of days off. The last thing I wanted would be to get injured now, that would be a disaster. But after resting for a few days I noticed I had become extremely apathetic towards running, so actually having a bit of a niggle was pretty convenient. I wondered if part of the apathy was actually complacency. I had just run forty-four miles over two days; surely I had this in the bag? What could go wrong now I thought? A worrying sense of déjà vu washed over me – that was pretty much what happened during my second Abingdon marathon attempt – I got complacent. It was a very dangerous thing to do, so I made a mental note to try and snap myself out of it. In the end I didn't run all week partly to give my ankle a good rest and partly because – in truth – I just couldn't really be bothered.

The following Sunday, now with only three weeks to go, I went out for a slow run from Warmley, heading out through the country lanes around Oldland Common and up towards Kelston. But as I ran up Redfield Lane, I reached the top of the hill and was struck by a pain in my head so violent it made me stop and grab onto a fence post to stop me from falling over. My vision blurred and I felt an overwhelming urge to vomit. The pain was sudden and intense and I stood there for what seemed like ages (although was probably only a few seconds) wondering what the hell was happening. Almost as quickly as the pain had come on it started to fade. I contemplated turning around and heading home, however I thought I would stroll for a bit first and if it seemed OK then I would just carry on. I had visions of being found in a ditch somewhere hours later after suffering a massive brain haemorrhage. After about five minutes of walking the pain seemed to have passed, so I cautiously carried on. I continued to run the rest of my planned route up to Kelston Round Hill, down to Weston on the edge of Bath and back to Warmley along the cycletrack. After having taken a week off I was hoping to feel refreshed but that turned out not to be the case. To top things off my ankle still wasn't quite right and I had developed a strain in my groin too, so I took it steady and made a mental note to call Dave Adler and get in and see him as soon as I could. Time was short now and I didn't want to screw it all up this late in the day. I already had an appointment booked back at the University of Bath on Tuesday to undergo my fit and fat tests again for the "after" to go with my "before", so I would go to that but figured I would try not to push it too hard.

I managed to get in and see Dave on Wednesday and explained to him that I thought I was starting to fall apart. His diagnosis was a problem with my peroneal tendon (which runs along the outside of the ankle) with *"an acute-on-chronic lateral ligament strain"*. He thought I had probably aggravated an old ligament injury, one probably caused from falling off my BMX so many times years before. He carried out a bit of ultrasound and some stretching and sent me on my way with some stretches to keep up with. I took it easy for the next week and whilst I can't say that the groin and ankle were perfect, they slowly faded away and I forgot about them. There were only a couple of weeks left to go now and I was getting nervous of doing myself any real damage. I wanted to lock myself in a cupboard until race day, just to stay safe, but that wasn't going to happen.

As the training was finally coming to a close I looked back over what I had achieved over the previous twenty or so weeks and I was amazed at how far I had come. I was slimmer; fitter; healthier and now had a real chance of actually pulling the whole thing off. The route had been memorised and seemed omnipresent. Whenever I drove around Bristol, I found myself spotting places where the Green Man route crossed roads and went over bridges. Overall I felt remarkably calm about the whole process and was looking forward to the upcoming weekend. Maybe I became a bit complacent with it all, which I tried very hard not to but I did feel confident. When you're such an optimist, it's often hard to feel anything else.

Talking to Bear though he wasn't quite as confident and was in fact quite worried by the prospect of the whole thing – the whole challenge of the unknown. What would it be like to run more than thirty miles in one go? How could a man who got lost in his own house manage to find his way all around Bristol? How are we even going to be able to stand on half marathon day? Was it all just a stupid idea?

With the Bath Half Marathon a mere matter of weeks away the publicity department at Macmillan Cancer Support went into overdrive and sent out various press releases to assorted local press, which subsequently saw a picture of me grinning widely after a recce run to Hambrook being featured in the Bath Chronicle. Somebody called me to tell me that I had also been on the radio in Bristol too talking about the weekend, which was certainly news to me. Whether or not it all garnered any interest remained to be seen but it was out there and it could certainly do no harm. I had already raised almost £1000 with money and pledges still coming in, all of which had exceeded my expectations already. All I had to do now was stay in one piece and actually run the bloody thing.

14. Can You Still Pinch an Inch?

"Beware of the pursuit of the Superhuman;
it leads to an indiscriminate contempt for the human."
– George Bernard Shaw

With the training at an end I headed back up to the University of Bath and the Human Performance Centre to run through the same set of tests I had undergone back at the start of October. This time around I was undoubtedly fitter and slimmer than I had been before but by just how much was the big question.

It had become quite apparent – even from my delusional perspective – that with my recent string of injuries, ailments and incidents that I was so very far from being either bionic or superhuman, but could all my focussed training and hard work have brought me up to the supreme levels of Karnazes et al? No of course it couldn't, that would require some kind of divine intervention, but as Max Ehrmann wrote in my favourite poem, Desiderata:

"If you compare yourself with others, you may become vain and bitter;
for always there will be greater and lesser persons than yourself."

Whatever the outcome of the retest I could only be happy with what I had already achieved and pleased that considering where I started I was now in a position to be able to seriously take on the challenge that lay ahead and hopefully finish without any serious problems.

Back at the university I met up with Jonathan once again in the small nondescript room overlooking the pool and stripped down to my underwear ready to be drawn on, measured and squeezed with the fat grapplers. Working down the right side as before Jonathan jotted down the required measurements to enable him to work out how fat I still was. Numbers taken I got dressed, jumped onto the treadmill and jogged for five minutes to warm up ready for the lactate and VO$_2$ max tests. Just like the last time, the treadmill test started with me running for three minutes at 8kph before jumping to the sides and having blood taken to test my lactate levels. Then after briefly catching my breath, the belt would speed up by 1kph and I would jump back on and go again. Repeat until collapse. The first time I did the test I managed to keep the efforts going up to 15kph (about six minutes and twenty-five seconds per mile) at which point I really couldn't run any further. This time however I still felt strong as I passed the same point and I pushed on through 16kph, to give what I would deem as a credible attempt at the next rep. At this point I had been running for twenty-four minutes at an ever increasing pace and I was just about to jump back onto a treadmill that was revolving at 17kph (five minutes and forty seconds a mile). In hindsight I never had a chance of completing that rep, but as I so often would, I jumped on anyway and gave it a good go. Perhaps what I should have done was get Jonathan to hook me up to the safety harness first to stop my face from being ground down by the spinning sander belt after my legs had collapsed beneath me but unfortunately that didn't cross my mind until it was too late. Initially my legs complied with my brain and I ran on, determined to get to the next level, but what I realised pretty quickly was that as explained by Einstein's theory of relativity, under certain circumstances time really can dilate and slow down. I had seemingly been running for minutes; hours; days even, when it had in fact been less than a paltry sixty seconds. Debating with myself whether to save face and call it, or to keep going, I battled with the urge to stop but ninety seconds in I knew I had no chance of making it to three minutes and staying upright, so I jumped to the sides and threw in the towel. It was a good effort, however I was beaten. Looking at the graph on the computer screen next to me measuring my breathing I could see I was well into oxygen deficit, meaning it would have been increasingly tough to keep going for much longer anyway. Given I hadn't really been training for speed it was a decent result. The key though would be the lactate and oxygen readings that would come out of the tests. Stepping down off the treadmill I was sweating profusely and had given it everything I had. The minor groin injury I had been nursing for the last week or so seemed to have disappeared which was welcome news although my ankle tweaked on the back-to-back weekend was still fairly sore. All of that aside, the second set of tests for comparison were done, now I just needed to sit back and wait for the results to roll into my inbox.

The very next day in came the email from Jonathan, complete with the detailed report from the tests. Opening the document up, I scanned straight through it for my fat figure. More than anything else I was curious how much fat I still had hanging around. I knew I had lost weight but also knew I wasn't super thin. I certainly wasn't a ten stone skeleton, in fact I was still just over fourteen – around two and a half stone down from when I ran the Bristol Half Marathon the September before and almost three lower than early 2012. It would have been nice to have dropped a bit more weight although already my mum was already telling me I looked gaunt (although I'm not sure she was looking at me) and I certainly didn't feel conscious of being fat anymore. In the first calliper test Jonathan calculated me as having a body fat percentage of 21.1%, which according to the WHO was somehow just about within the normal healthy range for a man of my age, this second time around however I had dropped that to just 13.1%. I was amazed. I knew I was slimmer but didn't quite expect it to be that low. It was a great result and testament to my abstention of cakes, pizza and beer. As before, the measurements showed that despite being the area that had reduced the most, the bulk of the blubber I had left still resided around my midriff, there was just less of it there.

I read on and looked up the results of the lactate and VO_2 max tests which also showed a marked improvement on the previous tests. While your absolute VO_2 max is exactly that – absolute, by dropping weight and improving fitness you can improve your relative score. For me, my previous was 48.0 ml/kg/min which was already pretty good, however the new and improved me clocked in with a new score of 52.7 ml/kg/min which put me firmly into the *"excellent"* bracket, above the ranges expected for a guy of my age. Jonathan added to the findings saying: *"VO_2 is lower across the range of speeds in Feb compared to Oct, thus you are using less oxygen to go at the same speed therefore you are more economical or efficient. This is an ideal adaptation for your chosen event."* Ideal indeed.

Moving onto the lactate results I analysed the threshold velocity, which is the first significant rise of blood lactate above the recorded baseline levels. Back in October it measured 163bpm/11kph which in itself again wasn't too bad, but at the retest that had moved up to 170bpm/12kph. What this meant in plain English was that I was able to run harder and faster for longer before the lactic acid build up really started to affect my performance. Plotted on a graph, the lactate data from February drew a much lower and flatter line than the previous test, which rose slower and later. This was very good news and physiologically exactly the result I was looking for based upon the heart rate zones I had been training within.

Jonathan closed the report with a statement that summed it all up nicely, saying: *"It is clear that for a standalone marathon or longer length performance, LT (lactate threshold), economy, and to a much lesser extent VO2 Max are the most important factors to consider, and from that statement it indicates improving your current LT and running economy will provide great benefits to you. The key therefore to improved performances is to improve LT and your running economy further. This has clearly occurred over the last few months and thus you have made the correct physiological adaptations for the event that you aim to complete. Well done you have clearly put in the right type of effort over the last 4 months."*

Overall the results were great. I had followed the scientific approach and it had delivered on its promise. Now together with feeling fitter, running better and being lighter, I also had the added weapon of psychologically knowing that science had proved me to be in good shape and ready to take on the ultramarathon weekend. It was precisely the outcome I was looking for. In the words of Hannibal Smith: *"I love it when a plan comes together"*.

15. The Calm Before the Storm

"If you think about racing too much you may just lose it a little bit."
– Usain Bolt

With just over a week to go, there really was nothing more to do. The training was finished, the retests were done and I wasn't going to be losing any more weight now. The last couple of weeks were all about tapering down and now into the final stretch, I had planned to scale down to more or less nothing. The best way to do as little as possible I figured was to jet away on holiday for the last week and lounge around in the sun. This needed some thought however, as to go somewhere warm in February meant spending more than a couple of hours on a plane but at the same time not venturing too far afield, as the last thing I needed was to be fighting jetlag whilst running all weekend. Looking through a few options, one ideal solution that jumped out was Lanzarote in the Canary Islands. Despite being under Spanish jurisdiction Lanzarote operates on the same time zone as the UK, meaning zero jetlag and sitting just off the coast of North Africa it was also warm all year round.

As is generally the case with charter flights to tourist islands such as the Canaries, they often only change over one day of the week from each regional airport and as it turned out the flights from Bristol were on a Thursday. What this meant was that I wouldn't get back to the UK until late the following Thursday, leaving just one day to spare before the weekend. It was a tad close for comfort. All it would take would be an air traffic controller strike or volcanic ash cloud to strand me on the island and I might not be able to get back in time for the weekend. After everything I'd been through to get to this point that would be a disaster. Nevertheless, I figured if it actually came down to that, it would actually make a great tale for the book – I could just run the races on my own after I got back and try and blag the medals from the race organisers afterwards.

Reading up on the resort of Playa Blanca where we were staying, I discovered there was a dormant volcano on the edge of the town which was a popular trail walk for tourists. I decided that running up it whilst I was there sounded like a nice challenge to drop into the week, just to ensure my legs were still working. After all the hill training over the winter I figured I was probably ready for a small volcano. That was until we arrived and I saw just how big it was in real life. Montaña Roja was hardly the largest volcano on the island, but no photos I had seen of it had actually done it justice. It certainly looked much larger and more impressive in real life than I had anticipated it to be. Driving by the base, I saw a chain of walkers making their way steadily along the trail that weaved up the side and around the rim. They looked like ants inching along the rocky path. Not wanting to chicken out on the idea, I decided to play safe and give myself a few days to "acclimatise to the temperature" (ie: talk myself into it) before taking it on.

Being February it wasn't as hot as it would have been in the peak of summer, although after the winter we had just experienced a balmy twenty-five degrees was luxurious. Falling foul of my optimism on the first day, I didn't bother with such piffling things as putting on sun block – *"don't worry, it's not that hot"* – and spent the bulk of the day poolside soaking up the sun and catching up on my reading. The next day I woke looking a distinctly brighter shade of pink. I dropped Bear a text message to see how he was preparing and apparently it was so cold back in Bristol he had gone polar and reverted to type, taking to hibernating for the week. I figured maybe being a little bit pink wasn't so bad after all.

Getting up on Saturday I decided it was a good day to take on a volcano. I was mentally prepared and if it was totally horrific I would still have a whole week to get over it. It was only going to be a short run, a few miles at most, but thought I should probably have some breakfast anyway. The trouble was while at home I would normally fuel up on a bowl of porridge or some other form of slow-release carbohydrates well suited to the demands of exercise but being on holiday we didn't have any such thing in the cupboards. In the end I ran on a generous helping of Golden Grahams. I'm not quite sure who Graham was, nor why he was golden but nevertheless he seemed to do the job just fine. Leaving the villa and heading off in the general direction of the volcano, I realised I didn't actually know where the path started. The enormous lump of rock sticking out the ground was a bit of a clue, as was the helpful sign I stumbled across stating *"Al Volcan"* (the volcano) was to the right. Far from looking like an official tourist office installation though, this was hand painted on an old plank and nailed to a wonky post. It looked more like it had been stuck up by someone fed up with groups of tourists traipsing through their back garden searching for a trail up a volcano. Following the sign around the corner I saw an arrow painted on a rock on the ground which in turn led me to the beginning of the trail. From the bottom I could see plenty of people making their way up the mountain, albeit walking slowly. Strewn with rocks the route was somewhat hazardous to run on, but skipping side-to-side past handfuls of walkers, I zigzagged my way up the hill, taking care where I placed my feet, ensuring I didn't do any further damage to my ankle that had only recently recovered.

The sun was shining and even though it was only around eight in the morning it was already pretty warm, all of which meant that by the time I reached the rim I looked as if I had stopped and taken a shower en-route, although I prefer to think of it as having an "athletic sheen" as opposed to just being wringing wet with sweat. In all honesty, despite appearing brutal and unforgiving from the bottom, the climb wasn't actually half as bad as I had envisaged. I couldn't decide if that was because it was in fact pretty easy or because I was running well, maybe all the hill training in Bath had paid dividends; either that or the volcano was just somewhat illusory in size. Looking at the GPS data afterwards it was actually a good six-hundred and fifty feet above sea level at the top – higher than any of the climbs I had run up in training (we walked up Dundry Hill), but it was still really more of a hill than a mountain to be fair. Regardless, I had conquered it and could now claim to have run up a bonafide volcano – even if it did sound much grander than it was in reality. I followed the trail around the rim, stopping for a few minutes on the far side to sit and look out over the water towards Fuerteventura. The view was incredible and had totally been worth the effort. I even managed to collar a random German walker coming the other way to take a few snaps of me as evidence I had made it to the top.

I spent the rest of the week largely lying around, floating in a pool, or reading – sometimes all at once. There was also a distinct lack of beer consumption over the span of the week, which was also something new to me whilst being on holiday. It felt slightly odd to be doing so little after having spent so much time running over the previous months. I did go out for a couple of easy three-mile jogs around the resort just to ensure my legs did still work, one of which ended with me being chased (but not caught) out of an exclusive gated complex. The training however was officially over.

In the end there was to be no air traffic controller strike, no ash cloud and no flight delay, all of which meant I arrived home as planned on Thursday evening, slightly more tanned than I had left and about as relaxed as I could be under the circumstances.

Over the previous twenty-two weeks I had run a shade over six-hundred and seventeen miles in training, making an average of

16. New Man vs. Green Man

*"Run when you can, walk if you have to, crawl if you must;
just never give up."* – **Dean Karnazes**

Rolling out of bed just after five o'clock on Saturday morning I wandered down to the kitchen where I had already laid out all my supplies for the coming day. The sugar-laden spread arranged in front of me looked like a diabetic's suicide dinner. There were energy gels; Snickers bars; fruitcake; chocolate-coated energy bars; jelly beans; and a few bottles of Powerade. I packed it all neatly into my backpack for the day together with the mandatory items of kit dictated by the race organisers. In the small bright orange ten-litre bag with my sugary treats went a compass; foil blanket; whistle; first aid kit; OS maps 155 and 167; mobile phone with GPS; and a headtorch complete with spare batteries. With that little lot packed and the two-litre drinks bladder topped up to full the bag was ready, if somewhat heavy. It all felt a little over the top for just another run but then again this wasn't just another run. This was it – the big one, the one it had all been about. Everything I had gone through over the last five or so months had been all for this day. Despite how well the training had gone and how ready I thought I was, I was packing a bag that needed to hold enough calories to sustain me as I ran close to fifty miles in one go. If it felt over the top then so be it, that's what it needed to be.

Watching my calorific intake for weight loss had gone well over the previous months and as I stood on the scales that morning I weighed in at a sporting 14st 1lb. It was still a long way from being slim but it was almost three stone down from my hefty peak the year before. Despite still not being a slight long-distance runner, it was certainly a positive result and one that had taken some effort to achieve. My body fat measurements from the Human Performance Centre report told me that the bulk of my remaining fat still resided around my middle and that would take much more focussed work to remove, but I had certainly transformed myself into reasonable fighting shape for the task at hand. The truth is I was still a tall and sizable guy. I was never going to be a ten stone waif and in truth I wouldn't want to be.

I sat at my dining table, fully dressed ready for the event, to a warming bowl of porridge garnished with a generous squirt of maple syrup and a couple of mugs of very strong coffee. As I ate I wondered how the day would pan out, more than anything else what kind of shape I would be in this time tomorrow. After my brief flirtation with an ice bath during our double run weekend I decided not to try that again. I figured I would take my chances with a bit of dinner and an early night. If I was feeling awake I might even take a warm dip with a touch of Radox. I was of course somewhat jumping the gun and working on the assumption that I was actually going to finish. There was still the small matter of running forty-six miles before I could run a bath.

Setting out from my house to the Redwood Hotel the weather showed signs of being kind for the day. Whilst it had been cold in recent weeks (and still was) it had also been much drier than it had been through our soggy months of training. It would still be muddy on the ground but if the sun was shining then it would make it all that much more bearable. With dawn still yet to break, I drove through the dark morning, diagonally across the city I was about to run a gigantic loop around and mentally prepared myself for the run. I went over the course in my head, ticking off each gate, hedge and stile as I visually made my way around the footpath. I was confident I knew the route but last-minute nerves were playing on those memories bringing the more unfamiliar parts into question.

Arriving at the hotel I parked up and walked into the gymnasium to collect my number from the ad-hoc race headquarters. It was still early although there were already a good handful of eager looking runners milling about inside, eating, stretching and pinning laminated race numbers to themselves. I met up with a nervous looking Bear and collecting our numbers we could see that our decision to both run clearly had an influence on each other at the time of registration as I was entrant number ten and Bear was eleven. Guy, who turned up shortly afterwards, clearly took a little more persuasion as he sported a lofty sixteen. Numbers pinned on and munching on a seed-based energy bar we took a few photos and had a little stroll around, bumping into Bill as he came in to register. He wasn't sure of how the day would pan out for him as he had been suffering from a foot injury and his training hadn't quite gone to plan, but he figured he had nothing to lose by turning up and giving it a good go anyway. Getting to the start line alone for long-distance events is almost as much of a challenge as completing them, with the risk of injury from overtraining being seriously high. I'd suffered my own share of niggles along the way but thankfully everything seemed to have settled down. We went for a walk around the car park and caught Lynette pulling up outside. Like Bill, she too wasn't sure how she would get on now it was actually race day. She confessed that she had struggled slightly whilst running the back-to-back weekend with us and was worried that she might suffer the same fate today, especially after passing out following a long bike ride only the week before. Having done all the training however she wasn't going to let a few last-minute nerves stop her now and wandered off into the gym to register and collect her race number.

Standing around outside I tried to get a good mobile signal

to enable me to post an update to my Facebook page, informing everyone who had sponsored me that I was here and ready. I had decided to post a few messages as I went to keep those interested updated with how the day was unfolding. This wasn't going to be a two-hour wait for a half marathon result, this was the best part of a whole day from dawn to dusk and naturally people would wonder how it was going. With patchy reception obtained, just before the start I managed to post a snap of Bear, Guy and myself smiling and raring to go. Comments of good luck came back almost instantly and the ball had started rolling. There really was no way back now.

With sunrise just before seven o'clock it was bright and sunny by the time the crowd of runners gathered at the back of the hotel just before eight. Men, women and dogs alike (there was also a Green Man canicross challenge), all stood ready for the off, listening as the race director gave us our final instructions for the day. In contrast to the start of pretty much every road race I had ever ran the mood amongst the seventy or so of us assembled was light-hearted and friendly – perhaps even jovial. Looking around me there were people of all ages, sizes and backgrounds yet it felt as if there was something unsaid connecting us, something shared, something communal. No doubt in the last six months most of us had been told by somebody that running forty-six miles was insane – maybe that's what we all had in common. Granted it certainly wasn't a normal way to spend a Saturday in early spring but standing in the starting pack waiting for the air-horn to be sounded I was excited, nervous and apprehensive, yet still strangely confident. Surely as an optimist it was impossible to be anything but?

As the clock struck eight and the horn sounded we were off. The pack, all grouped together, ran out the back of the hotel, past a pair of distinctly icy-looking swimming pools and turned left onto a gravel path that ran down towards the red deer enclosure. This first section of the route was one that we hadn't bothered recceing given that at the start there would be plenty of people around and at the end it should be familiar from only having run it earlier in the day. Nice logic, but whether it would match reality we would have to wait and see.

The trail to Ashton Court took up almost the first couple of miles and what we didn't notice as we all ran down it far too fast fired up for the day, was that it was actually a decent downhill gradient – great for a quick start although painful for finishing with forty-four miles already in your legs. The cheery and relaxed nature of the pack carried through with jokes rolling and laughter rippling with energy through the huddled runners as we all grouped together to pass through the first kissing gate one at a time. Once inside the enclosure the group thinned out as people made their break and set their own pace for the day. We followed the path down through the familiar pay and display car park where we had abandoned our cars a number of times in training only weeks before and whisked by the mansion house, through the adjoining field and out past The Dovecote pub on the edge of the estate. Passing the Park and Ride site we now ventured onto the first really muddy section that ran between the A370 Long Ashton bypass and the even more major A38. The ground was still boggy – although nothing like it had been the first time we had been here. It was enough to slow a number of runners down and allow the pack to spread out even further. By this time we had already lost sight of the leaders, as well as Bill and Lynette who seemed to tag along with him. I wondered if considering her concerns after the training, that setting off at such a rapid pace was a wise move for her but only time would tell.

Bear, Guy and I had originally all planned to run the race together. We told ourselves that it wasn't about the time, it was about the endurance; it was about completing it; about becoming ultramarathon runners. This plan came into question however when in the last weeks of training it became apparent that Bear struggled a little more than Guy and myself over some of the more difficult terrain and didn't feel as confident at being able to run the kind of pace dictated by the time we had originally pencilled in – sub ten hours. We had a conversation about it the week before where we discussed that despite the fact that he wasn't as self-assured as me, I was still happy to stick to our plan to run together. Just because I was feeling strong (which could have simply been a fatal combination of training and delusion) I wasn't suddenly going to abandon him and run off into the sunset. The Rolf Harris tune *"Two Little Boys"* came into my head, before being flushed quickly out again. Bear said he would be happy with either approach. He didn't want me to hamper my own race by waiting around for him as had happened a couple of times on training runs but at the same time if I was happy to run slower with him then that too would be fine.

It presented me with a difficult decision and I was somewhat torn. On one hand I felt I should stick to our original idea and run it together. That is what we had agreed. We signed up together, trained together and we would finish together. On the other hand however, whilst Bear was confident of finishing, he wasn't anywhere near as confident as I was of doing so in less than ten hours. He figured he could be as much as an hour adrift of that target. With that kind of window of time between the two we decided to all set out together and so long as nobody was too far behind then we would stick together but if somebody dropped back well out of sight or was clearly struggling then the others should push on. It wasn't a race that any of us was ever going to win and irrespective of time we would all be awarded a medal anyway. All that said you always want to cross that finish line feeling like you had done your very best. It was the only way to do all your training justice.

Crossing the A38 and diving up behind the Town and Country Lodge, we ploughed through an assortment of churned up fields taking us to the bottom of Dundry Hill, where as planned we dropped to a walking pace and hiked up to the transmitters. It was a steep climb that didn't get any easier with familiarity but after a swift start it was good to slow the pace and take the opportunity to snack as we walked. From the top we ran down the wide gravel trail to the large gate that led us into Dundry village, where the three of us met Jon waiting with a flask of hot coffee. We stopped briefly and swigged back the warm caffeine, taking in the incredible view across Bristol from such a high vantage point. A quick chat about how it was going and off we set again, down through the handful of fields and farms that followed, taking us into Norton Malreward and the first checkpoint at just under ten miles.

With our goal being to finish in less than ten hours I had calculated a rough plan with timings to reach each checkpoint, so we could see how we were faring against our target. Our predicted time of arrival at the first checkpoint was to be just after ten o'clock but as we rolled into the village hall and checked in it was still only nine forty-five – a good fifteen minutes up on our agenda. Whilst this was good news, it was also worthy of caution making sure we hadn't set out too fast and were tiring ourselves too quickly. Stopping to refuel on whatever snacks I had in my bag and stuff that was laid out for us I posted my first Facebook update from the run: *"Checkpoint 1 – Norton Malreward. 9:45. Feeling good. Cashback!"* Still all together, we rested at the checkpoint for about five minutes before pushing on through the churchyard, over the tiny airfield and down into Pensford. Running through the village we met up with a fellow Bitton Road Runner, Chris Brown, who had timed his Saturday morning run to catch us on our way and he joined us for a couple of miles as we ran through Woollard (dodging the same large bull in the same small field as before), heading towards the second checkpoint.

Running through Compton Martin towards Keynsham it was clear how much drier the whole path was. It was amazing how much the water levels had receded and how firm the ground had become over only a matter of a few weeks. With a little less squidge underfoot, it certainly made the going that little bit easier. At this point, following the river down towards town there was still a good number of runners both in front and behind us, which was strangely comforting. It was reassuring to know both that we were still on the right path and that we weren't running so slowly as to make fools of ourselves. Carrying on along the river, passing through Keynsham Park we soon found ourselves arriving at the Lock Keeper Pub and checkpoint two. It was just over seven miles on from the first checkpoint and we had now covered around seventeen miles in total. Waiting at the checkpoint for us were Scott, Fay and Helen from work, as well as Phil, all of whom had made the special trip purely to cheer us on. Seeing so many friendly and supportive faces gave us a lift and we stood around and had a bit of a natter as we stuffed our faces with cake, gels and sweets grabbed from the collection of food laid out under the official race gazebo.

We were now just over a third of the way around the path and feeling pretty good about it all. The air was still good-humoured and we were loving every minute of it. I whipped out my phone, took a few snaps and posted my second update: *"Checkpoint 2 done. 11:05. 30 minutes up. Boom!"* At this point Bear had dropped back a little from Guy and me, turning up at the checkpoint about five minutes behind us, as we were getting ready to leave. As we set out on the next section, we left him there chatting and refuelling. What we didn't know at the time was that it would turn out to be the last time we would see him until the finish (a fact exacerbated by his getting hopelessly lost shortly afterwards and adding a couple of miles to his day).

The section of the Community Forest Path between Keynsham and the third checkpoint at The White Horse pub in Hambrook was very familiar territory to me as it had been the chunk I had run the most, as well as being the part of the path closest to my house. We took the path following the river through Willsbridge and joined onto the Bristol to Bath cycletrack before taking the dramway path to Warmley. Running on firm tarmac after so many miles in mud was quite a novelty, although it did highlight the fact that I had developed a blister on the sole of my right foot. It didn't feel too bad although I certainly wasn't going to take my mud-caked trainers off now and tend to it. My plan was to just plough on and try to ignore it. Emerging from the end of the lane that took us onto the main A420 we were greeted by a cheery group of Bitton Road Runners who had come out to help us along. We stopped for a quick chat before inching down the road to the old station to meet up with my wife and kids who had also ventured down to offer their support. We were around twenty miles in at this point and still feeling strong, yet to feel the real pains of tiredness, although things were starting to tighten up a little. Leaving the family behind we ran on up through Shortwood, past the creepy house in the woods and around the enormous landfill site, taking us back onto another stretch of cycletrack close to Pucklechurch. By this point we were pretty much halfway and starting to stiffen up we decided to stop for some food and a bit of a stretch. Taking my backpack off to pull out a handful of cake, I posted a midpoint update to Facebook: *"Halfway in 4:35. We're taking this puppy home now. Mine's a pint. Loving it."* The mental hurdle of reaching the halfway point was both exciting and daunting at the same time. We were now fifty percent of the way there. Every step we now took would mean we had covered more ground than we had left to run. Despite still having twenty-three miles to run, it felt as if we were closing down the distance to the finish. Needless to say we were both beginning to feel the miles we had already done and after four and a half hours of running it would be naïve to think we wouldn't be. We had pretty much just run a marathon and as I munched down a chunk of fruit cake, we laughed

Looking around I was surprised to see Bill at the checkpoint and went over for a quick chat. As it turned out his recent foot injury had flared back up and he had been forced to pull out of the race. He had opted to drop out at Hambrook strategically as it was the closest point to his house. He gave me a bit of a pep talk and reiterated the fact that we were doing well although the next bit was where it was going to start getting tough. We were about to enter into unknown territory, having only run as far as this once during training. In my head, this was where the real challenge started. I knew I could run twenty-eight miles in one go, I'd done that before but past that how far could I keep it up? With stiff legs, sugary teeth and a tired brain, we set off in the general direction of Bradley Stoke, my extreme optimism trying to continue to put a smile on it all. There was just over ten miles to the next checkpoint, and it was – in my mind – the toughest section of the footpath, with some steep hills and soulless fields of mud to tackle.

The biggest novelty of this section of the route came when we reached the motorway crossing over the M5 in Patchway, as the new bridge was actually completed and open. It was just as well, because the state we were in by that point there was no way I would have been able to not climb a security fence again. Dropping down the rocky gully into Easter Compton we plodded on, seemingly through field after field. As me and Guy talked we laughed at the absurdity of the whole thing. By this time we had been on our feet and largely running for nearly eight hours, which is longer than I would normally sit at my desk at work each day. Yet we were still going. Sure we had slowed down and the pack of runners had thinned out so much by now that it was rare to come across anybody else. We walked our way up the horrific climb that was Spanorium Hill, through the fields that followed, crossed back over the M5 and into Henbury. Once again back on tarmac we hobbled our way slowly through the housing estate and towards our final checkpoint before the end, checkpoint four at the Blaise Inn.

We ambled into the car park and slumped into hard plastic garden chairs that despite their lack of softness were absolutely luxurious. We were fast becoming exhausted but we hadn't finished yet. There was still the small matter of another eight miles to go. We had lost a chunk of our time in hand but our sub ten hour target was still a reality if we could keep moving at a steady pace. Talking to the marshals at the checkpoint they told us that the race leader, Darryl Carter, had been through there at a little after one-thirty – an hour in front of the runner in second place. To put this into perspective, we arrived at just after four o'clock. It was a staggering performance that we couldn't quite take in with our tired brains. As I munched on handfuls of sweets and cereal bars I posted my final checkpoint Facebook update: "*Checkpoint 4. 16:05. Still 10 minutes up on our plan, with about 8 miles to go. Pretty certain I've lost one toenail on my left foot. A little tired (mostly of running) but OK. Gonna smash this last stage in the face, steal its dinner money, and spend it on beer.*" I was unsure as to the state of my toenail however it certainly didn't feel right; neither did the blister that felt like it had engulfed the sole of my right foot. Regardless of all of that though, we were nearly there. As we sat lounging in white plastic garden furniture in a pub car park, our tired legs pleased for the rest, we knew that irrespective of how shattered we felt or how slow we would be, at that point we knew the end was within our reach. We had already run close to forty miles and whilst the idea of another seven or eight wasn't cheery, it was nothing in the grand scheme of things. A smile crossed my face as I shovelled in another handful of cola bottles, because right there and then I knew that we were going to do it.

Aching and moaning we left the chairs behind and plodded off through Blaise Castle Estate in search of the elusive steps through the woods, which we eventually found more through luck than judgement. We ran down the clearing between the trees, crossing the green iron bridge and down over our final golf course of the day in Shirehampton. The next section of the route up through Stoke Bishop towards Clifton was largely uphill and true to our plan we gladly walked a large part of it. In fact it was only as Durdham Downs came into sight and the ground levelled out that we launched ourselves into a slow jog across the grass in the general direction of the Clifton Suspension Bridge.

Isambard Kingdom Brunel's bridge is without doubt one of the most iconic sights in Bristol, almost to the point that I think it can seem like something of a cliché but that afternoon it was a glorious sight to behold as it came into view. It was half-past five, the sun was still up and with around two miles left to run we jogged over the bridge safe in the knowledge that we could almost walk the rest of the way and still finish within our ten hour goal. I felt ecstatic – knackered but ecstatic. We had been running for nine and a half hours and the end was almost literally in sight. As we crossed over the bridge we caught up to another group of runners and we ran along together for a short distance, but knowing I was safe within my ten hour window, as they started to pull away – Guy with them – I just let them all go. I was perfectly happy to finish this last mile on my own.

The long downhill gravel trail that had led to such a fast start did indeed come back to haunt me as I attempted to climb it back to the finish. Checking my watch and seeing I still had time to spare I ambled my way up the hill until it levelled out once more where I picked the pace back up to a jog. Slowly and surely I closed off the last chunks of the route and as I came up on the rear entrance to the hotel, I saw my good running buddy Julian waiting there to cheer me in and jog in the last few hundred metres alongside me. As I turned back into the grounds and saw the icy looking swimming pools I had left behind so many hours before, I picked up my pace to get it over and done with. It felt like I was sprinting but I'm sure it was a little more than a hobble. Rounding the corner I spied the open gymnasium doorway and gave my legs the final surge of energy they needed. As I entered the building everyone inside clapped and cheered my arrival which only compounded my emotion at finishing. I had done it. I looked down at my GPS that confirmed I had run just over forty-six miles in 9 hours 48 minutes, a result which placed me thirty-seventh out of sixty finishers. I stopped, knowing that I didn't have to run any further and sat down. Feeling slightly overwhelmed by the whole thing, I got up again, walked over to the desk and collected my medal, t-shirt and certificate, before turning around and walking back out to my car to sit down again in comfort. I pulled out my phone and posted my final Facebook update of the day: *"And relax. 46.5 miles battered into the ground in 9 hours 48 minutes. Guy ran 9:43, and Rudi is still out there, about an hour behind. Many thanks for all the support and donations today. It's been amazing. Shattered now and having a little happy emotional sob in my car. Next up, Bath Half in the morning. Hmmm...."*

As it turned out despite getting lost Bear came in just eight places behind me in 10 hours 39 minutes, looking suitably exhausted – although to be fair he did run a couple more miles than we did. Also milling around at the finish was Lynette, who at the start of the day was worried how well she would get on. Pretty well as it turns out, coming in seventh place, placing first female in a time of 8 hours 3 minutes, setting a new female course record. The male course record was also broken by the returning champion, Darryl Carter, who smashed his own previous record by over thirty minutes, finishing in a staggering 6 hours 35 minutes. That's somewhere in the region of eight and half minutes per mile – for forty-six miles. An incredible performance.

The day had been amazing and all of the hard work of the previous winter had been worthwhile. On the day the event organisation was slick, the checkpoints well stocked and managed and the atmosphere among the runners had been like nothing I had ever experienced at any other race. The day had perhaps unsurprisingly been hard work; yet fun at the same time. As Bill had told me months before, it was all so very different to road running and dare I say it, actually quite a lot of fun overall.

Back in the hall and after polishing off a sizable plate of piping hot chilli con-carne and rice I hobbled off to the gym to scrounge a towel to take a shower. Where I had been sat around in the hall for some time the laces of my trainers had solidified with dried mud making them very hard to undo with fingers that didn't work. I contemplated getting into the shower wearing them although thought better of the idea. I stripped off my muddy clothes and stood under the hot soothing shower for what seemed like ages without having to move. It was a luxury. My legs were stiff and my feet were sore but I didn't really want to bend over to look at the damage just yet. That could wait until the morning.

Stepping out of the shower I spotted a set of scales, so I thought I would weigh myself. To my astonishment, despite eating all day and drinking the best part of four litres of water, I had actually lost six pounds over the course of the day. Not ideal, particularly if it was through dehydration. I made a mental note to ensure I drank plenty for the rest of the day.

I got dressed and after saying my goodbyes to everyone walked back to my car. I sat there for a moment feeling pleased with what I had achieved. I knew I had to run again tomorrow but felt I had done the day and all of the sponsorship money justice. I checked my phone for messages and scanned Facebook for comments and feedback. What I read however knocked the wind out of my sails. Just one hour before I had finished the race Remo had posted an update of his own: *"Having completed my latest 3 cycles of chemotherapy at the Royal Marsden Hospital I had my assessment scans on Wednesday to see how things are going. So far every scan has revealed that my cancer is getting worse, but since starting my latest round of treatment at the RMH in December my appetite has improved and I have had a lot of good days and so my expectations were high. No such luck though. Whilst my primary cancer in the oesophagus has shrunk (which is good), the secondary cancer in my liver has worsened to the point that no further chemotherapy or other treatment is planned. Many thanks for all your support which is hugely appreciated – I will keep you updated."*

The end of Saturday was tinged with sadness with such heart-breaking news. After my tears of joy of finishing the ultramarathon, came a few tears of sadness at such a tragic situation. It made me all the more determined on Sunday to do the best I could to finish the challenge I had undertaken and to raise as much money for Macmillan Cancer Support as I possibly could.

17. It's Not Over Yet

"Only those who will risk going too far can possibly find out how far they can go." – **T.S. Eliot**

Saturday night wasn't exactly the best night's sleep I'd ever had. Despite being worn out after a somewhat busy day, the fact that I had a largely detached flapping toenail on my left foot meant that as I rolled about in bed it kept catching on the duvet and waking me up with short stabs of pain. Obviously what I should have done was stick it down with something but by bedtime I wasn't capable of clear thought. Following on from the Facebook posts the day before I thought I'd start the day as I'd ended the previous one, with a brief update: *"Just rolled out of bed and feeling a little stiff, but to be honest I've felt worse. Got one toenail hanging off and two sizable blisters, all of which need taping up before the start at 11:00. Not hoping for too much today, survival would be fine. Good luck to everyone running in Bath today."* My gut instinct was that today was going to be a slow plod of a run. I was confident of getting around – I mean it was only a poxy thirteen miles – although it certainly wasn't going to be in any kind of rapid time. Survival would indeed be acceptable.

I sat down at the dining table once again ready for breakfast, only didn't have much of an appetite. I still had a myriad of energy gels and bars in my bag from the day before but couldn't stomach the thought of any of those, so I settled on a couple of pieces of toast and a strong coffee instead. I knew I would have to try to eat more to get through the day but with an eleven o'clock start there was plenty of time for munching to come.

I turned my attention to the war wounds incurred the day before and tried to decide how best to tackle them. With one loose toenail and two blisters to address I reached for my magic roll of silver duct tape and cut off two small strips. I wrapped the first around the loose nail and the second, placed over the freshly lanced blister on the adjacent toe. Then taking a longer wide piece of tape, I wrapped it all the way around my foot ensuring the blister below was sealed off from the outside world. My remedial wound dressings might have made my foot look like a cheap robot repair but so long as they protected me for the next few hours then they would be just fine. Getting the tape off again might prove problematic but I figured I'd deal with that as and when the problem occurred.

Repairs made, I got in my car and drove the familiar ten miles over to Bath, meeting up with everyone from work who was also running that day. Just as the day before, the weather was chilly with clear skies, ideal running conditions. All the team were there including Scott, Fay and Rebecca ready for the culmination of their winter training. For many it was to be their first half marathon and the nerves were clear and present. Guy and Bear were also there, both looking as weary as I felt, which made me feel a little better, knowing it wasn't just me suffering. Being honest I didn't feel too bad, sure my legs were stiff but as I alluded to in my Facebook message I had been in worse states after much shorter races.

We all wandered over to the Recreation Ground where the runners' village was located to get ready to leave our bags in the baggage tent. In stark contrast to the handful of runners the day before, here there were thousands of people milling around, moving between the various tents that were spread around the large ground. Bath Half Marathon is always a popular race with its fairly flat course and ideal timing in the run up to the London Marathon and in recent years it had grown in size even more turning it into one of the larger events on the half marathon calendar with over ten thousand runners taking part. The paradox of the event however is the fact that despite Bath is a UNESCO World Heritage Site, the two-lap course doesn't really take in any of the major features or sights of the city, in fact five miles of the route is made by running down the somewhat industrial and rather soulless Lower Bristol Road, which as far as I'm aware doesn't feature too heavily on the international tourist trail.

I strolled over to the Macmillan Cancer Support tent to meet up with the fundraising team and had a quick chat with Sadie Moore about how the weekend was going. She wished me the best of luck for the day and told me to come back afterwards to make sure I took advantage of the free massage service for their team. It certainly sounded like a good idea. I tried to catch up with Phil too who was also running however the sheer volume of people around put paid to that idea, despite that fact that he was dressed in a full body Dalek costume and shouldn't have been too tricky to spot. I handed over my stuff at the bag drop, wished the best to everyone else and walked through to join the thousands of others in the starting pens on Great Pulteney Street. As I stood in the pack waiting for the race to start I had no real idea how the next few hours were going to pan out. Even if I had to walk it I was determined to finish, although I hoped it wasn't going to come down to that.

The air-horn sounded and the huddle slowly edged forward over the constantly beeping chip timing mat, moving at a shuffle until everyone had just enough space to break free into a run and set off on their own personal challenge. Once the crowd had started moving the initial few steps were slightly painful and felt a bit clunky as if I was running with splints but within half a mile everything seemed to feel as if it had stretched out and I picked up the pace to a natural rhythm. Before I knew it I had covered the first mile in just over eight minutes and a small thought flickered in my delusional brain that maybe I could keep this pace going and run finish in around 1 hour and 45 minutes, which would be an awesome achievement, but as I came towards of the end of the second mile the degradation of my pace had already made my dream look extremely unlikely. I reminded myself that the goal of today was survival and not trying to run a good time. I would never be able to come close to my personal best time anyway, so easing off the speed and ensuring I finished was the only sensible option.

The first lap around was pretty uneventful as runs go and went by in something of a blur. Whether that was because I was now conditioned to running further or whether I was just in a bit of a daze I couldn't tell. I ran through the halfway point at 57 minutes which was faster than I was expecting and it spurred me on to think that running sub 2 hours was still a possibility. It was only a loose goal for sure and one that wasn't important but it was good to have a focus to keep me going. The whole experience in Bath was proving to be worlds apart from the mud and fields of the day before. Whereas on the Community Forest Path there were huge sections where Guy and I didn't see another runner, here I was constantly surrounded by them. Sometimes it's good to have company and crowds to cheer you on but sometimes all you want is to get your head down and run in solitude, without the crowds; without the cheering; without the bands and sound systems. Maybe that was just me being something of a miserable bastard at heart.

It wasn't until I got to about mile eight as I was passing Royal Victoria Park for the second time that I really began to flag. Over the span of about a mile I had really started to feel tired, maybe in part through my lack of food that morning but more likely just the combination of everything that had gone before. I slowed to a bit of a shuffle as I passed the park, clearly looking to be in some difficulty and a fellow charity runner pulled up alongside me to deliver some words of encouragement: "*Well done Macmillan, keep it going you're doing great."*, I responded without really thinking with *"Thanks dude, but I'm shattered. I think yesterday is catching up with me"*. It was a little more information than I really wanted to give away but with the unthinking slip of the tongue it was out there. I didn't want to have the conversation about the fact that I had ran an ultramarathon the day before, as it would be hard to do without sounding like I was boasting but alas it was too late.

"Oh you should have rested yesterday, what did you get up to?" At that point I didn't know if I should just tell him the truth or spin some tale to get him off my back. He was only trying to be supportive and help me along and I really didn't want to piss on his fire of help. With my tired brain unable to spin a viable yarn I instinctively decided honesty was probably the best policy.

"I ran forty-six miles in an ultramarathon around Bristol."

"You ran what?" His voice sounded slightly incredulous.

"All the way around Bristol, in a race. Yesterday."

His run hiccupped as if he missed a step and unsure if I was telling the truth or not, he looked at me for a second before retorting with a generic answer equally suited to either a lie or a truth: *"F**k off!"* As he pulled away I decided not to hold any more conversations during the run.

Keeping my pace steady I jogged along at around a ten minute mile pace. I was unsure whether or not I was still going to make the sub 2 hour window I had set myself up for but as I turned back onto the Lower Bristol Road and the long home straight it was still a distinct possibility. I sauntered down the wide road counting down the miles left till I could stop. Waves of tiredness were washing over me now and my legs were beginning to get very heavy. I went through mile nine, then ten and eleven. The finish was so nearly within my grasp but as I went through the twelve mile mark (or fifty-nine as I like to think of it) it felt like somebody took a cricket bat to the back of my legs. All the strength and power went out of them and despite a desperate urge to keep running I gave in and began to walk. I say walk, to be honest it was more of a hobble. It was at this point that Bill's words rang back through my head: *"Just keep moving – at any speed."* It made sense, although slow was the speed I was thinking of.

I limped my way past the end of North Parade with less than half a mile to go, runner after runner telling me to keep going because we were nearly there. I blocked them out as I walked, they had no way of knowing what I'd been through over the last couple of days and whilst their encouragement was friendly and well-intentioned it wouldn't bring my legs back to life. I told myself that I should run the finishing straight on Pulteney Street where it had begun earlier in the day, so I should save my energy for that. Coming up on the final corner I looked at my watch which helpfully informed me that I had already gone over the two-hour mark I had hoped to get under but I didn't care. As I set out at the beginning of the day the sole aim was simply completion. Just over two-hundred metres now stood between me and that. I turned the corner and willed my dead legs into action and ran as fast as my exhausted body would allow, shouting obscene motivation to myself. As I ran down the wide road lined with cheering spectators, I stumbled over the timing mat hitting the stop button on my watch as I did so. I stood for a brief second making sure I hadn't missed something and somebody was going to tell me to keep moving. But nobody said anything, I was done. I had completed the half marathon in 2 hours 6 minutes – the very same time it took me to finish my very first half marathon thirteen years earlier – and with that I had completed the weekend and the challenge. After months of talking, planning and training, it was over.

Tired, happy and slightly emotional I walked through the crowd collecting my medal and goody bag and made my way back to the Macmillan Cancer Support tent for a massage. It was heavenly and without doubt the single most important thing that enabled me to keep moving for the rest of the day. I met up with Scott and Bear afterwards we walked into town for some lunch and sat discussing the day and looking up everyone else's results.

Fay completed her very first half marathon in a commendable time of 2 hours 50 minutes only months after not being able to even run a mile. Bear finishing the weekend strongly with a time of 2 hours 20 minutes and Guy ran a staggering 1 hour 45 minutes exceeding all of our expectations. Rebecca had a great run too and smashed her previous best time by seven minutes to finish in a respectable 1 hour 41 minutes and Scott also ran a sterling race to finish in 1 hour 37 minutes, not quite a personal best but a great run nonetheless. The result of the day for me however was the Dalek I couldn't find at the start, Phil, who exterminated the competition finishing in a stellar 1 hour 25 minutes.

It had been a successful day and a grand conclusion to what had seemed only months before like an epic and unsurmountable challenge. The question now was where do you go from here?

18. Aftermath

"You must listen to your body. Run through annoyance but not through pain." – **George Sheehan**

It was finally all over – time to put my feet up and have a nice cup of tea, or even a cheeky cold beer. I had achieved what I had set out to do from the off: I was slimmer, fitter, eating healthier, drinking less and had just run a ridiculous amount of mileage over two days raising over £1400 for a good cause. It was a satisfying feeling to have completed it but now it was time to rest. There is some thinking that says to recover fully you need to rest one day for each mile you race, in this case that would mean taking the best part of the next two months off and there was no way I could see that happening. After pushing myself to the limit, I was amazed at how reasonable a shape I was still in. I could still walk, albeit a bit like C-3PO in a tar pit however I was still moving. The only physical damage I had amassed over the weekend was the loss of two toenails from my left foot and a sizable blister on my right. Being honest the run had only caused one of the nails to drop off, while the toe next to it had developed a large blister around the nail. It was only when I decided to undergo a little bathroom surgery late on Tuesday night I discovered it actually went right under the nail, and then that one became detached too. Being a bit obsessive I decided I had to sort them both out right away and so hacked away at the dead skin and nail beds with an old pair of rusty nail scissors until they looked like something out of a zombie movie. When I'd finished I looked down and knew I'd gone too far, because even I thought they looked disgusting. I dressed them as best as I could with a squirt of Savlon cream, some Andrex and a roll of Sellotape and went to bed. It was only when I got up in the morning and explained to my medically trained wife what I had done that I realised I had probably got a bit too carried away and now needed to get them seen to properly. I think *"bloody idiot"* was the phrase she used. So that lunchtime I hobbled into an NHS walk-in centre in Bath and saw a very helpful nurse who looked at me strangely as I entered the treatment room. I explained to her about my weekend and how my toes had come to be in such a state, when she said: *"That's where I know you from, I saw your picture in the Chronicle last week."* I was a celebrity. As she cleaned and dressed my self-inflicted wounds all she wanted to hear about were my ultramarathon exploits and I was more than happy to regale her with anecdotes of miles aplenty. After she'd finished I thanked her for her understanding of my butchery and I shuffled slowly back to work. As I did so I smiled to myself, thinking if this was the only damage I was coming away from this ultramarathon madness with then it was all good. I had garnered more injuries from much lesser runs, like the time one of my front teeth fell out during a Sunday morning run. It was actually only a post crown but even so it wasn't ideal timing, especially seeing as one of my contact lenses popped out at the same time – I was blind and toothless in the middle of the street. Or the time I was warming-up for the Clevedon 10K and gashed my head open running into a tree. I ran casually back the race headquarters with blood running down my face to looks of horror from the other runners. I'd never seen a first-aider gag before but to be fair it probably looked much worse than it was. After the race organiser gave me my entry fee back (probably just to get rid of me) I ended up in Frenchay Hospital having the meaty flap stuck back down with superglue and three stitches sewn around the edges to hold it down. But if they were both from mere jogs, getting

I'd enjoyed the handicap challenge races back in January and the sub nineteen minute 5K the month before, running fast was fun; exhilarating and those successes were all achieved off the back of just weight loss and improved fitness, without any real speed training. So I decided it was time to step back the distance, step up the speed and go for a fast half marathon. With a personal best of 1 hour 32 minutes, my target would have to be to run a sub 1 hour 30 minutes half marathon, which would be a very respectable time. Somehow however it didn't quite seem enough. Here I was at the peak of my fitness; I could do better than that. Why not target sub 1 hour 20 minutes I thought? Would that be so hard? Running six minute miles all the way around – that wasn't going to be easy, not unless I could get my old bionic legs back into service. But if I had proved anything with my training for the Green Man it was that I can achieve great things if I focused and worked hard. So it was that Operation 119 was born. My new plan was to run a half marathon in 1 hour 19 minutes. I printed out a poster and stuck it on the wall by my desk and I emailed several of my friends informing them of my new goal, at the Chippenham Half Marathon in September. Many of them scoffed openly in my face; however Bill and Phil, who had both run that fast in previous years, had faith that with focus I could do it. That was all the endorsement I needed. It was time to get fast.

I re-joined the gym, not because I had become a gym fan but if my 5K challenge had taught me anything it was that having the ability to go and run fast whatever the weather and with other people around was a huge boon. When it came to short sharp speed reps, a treadmill can prove extremely useful. It was exciting and all going so well, even if it was still early days.

At the start of this book I said that you never know what your body has genetically scheduled for you. Life is unpredictable and even if you could know what ailments or diseases you might contract, you'd still never know what accidents might befall you, or how external factors would affect your health and wellbeing. When I started this process I was fat, unfit and lazy. The optimist in me kept my attitude towards my health and wellbeing apathetic, assuming things were always just going to be alright, regardless of what I did. Then came the slap in the face – a friend diagnosed with a terminal illness that could have so easily been me. It gave me a kick up the ass and instilled a drive in me to get into better shape and care about my body and my health and it worked. However isn't it always the way that once you reach a good place, something comes along to smack you back down?

It was the morning after the lethargic run with Bear and I was driving to work as normal when I began to feel my left arm start to tingle. The sensation was odd, like sudden pins and needles from shoulder to fingertips. I initially dismissed it and thought if it still felt the same when I got in the office I'd look at it. A couple of minutes later and the left hand side of my face also began to tingle and go numb. Thinking this was now far from normal I pulled the car over and deliberated on calling 999 but it didn't really seem like ambulance material, so instead I looked up the number and called NHS Direct. After asking me half a dozen questions performing a quick telephone triage, they instructed me to get to a hospital as quickly as I could and tell them about our telephone conversation. I was quite close to the Royal United Hospital (RUH), on the outskirts of Bath, so I drove there, parked up in the car park and headed straight for A&E. As I started walking I noticed my left leg was also now tingling and numb. A quick conversation with the receptionist and I was ushered straight in, past the Monday morning crowd and a doctor was with me within a matter of minutes. It was certainly the fastest I'd ever been seen in a hospital. That *Chronicle* article had really got me known. He asked me a few questions, similar to the telephone triage and then informed me that he thought I could be having a stroke. I guess inside that's what I was thinking too, nonetheless to hear somebody else say it out loud was a shock. He immediately inserted a cannula into my arm and administered some drugs I didn't catch the name of. In the many hours that followed I had a CT scan of my head, a range of blood tests and saw two other doctors. Whilst the blood results and CT scan all came back clear, because of the continuing paraesthesia and numbness I was admitted to the Acute Stroke Unit, for me to undergo an MRI scan the following morning and to be assessed by the stroke consultants. A combination of never having spent the night in hospital, coupled with being wired up to a heart monitor and the fact I could have had some kind of stroke meant I didn't get a whole lot of sleep that night. I drifted in and out, but with wires stuck all over me my movement and my ability to get comfortable, was somewhat limited.

Morning rolled around and after a serving of Weetabix, tea and cold toast I was slid into an MRI scanner whilst listening to Johnny Cash singing *Ring of Fire* in a futile bid to drown out the clanging of the scanner making an image of the inside of my head. Back on the ward I was later visited by two stroke consultants who, after some questioning, decided I should also be examined by the neurological registrar. So after the best part of the day had passed, a third doctor came strolling in, looked me over, asked me the same handful of questions and went over to consult with the two other doctors. What followed next would best be described as a heated debate between the three, over their thoughts on my diagnosis. After the sparring had finished and the neurological registrar had left, I called one of the consultants back over who confirmed there was indeed a difference of opinion. The stroke consultants thought I had probably suffered some form of migraine, whereas the neurological registrar – who was a migraine specialist – thought it was more likely to have been a stroke. Cue another night on the ward so I could undergo a chest x-ray and ultrasound scans of my neck and left leg. Still, on the plus side, I was getting three meals a day for free and a pudding after dinner, which I never had at home. It wasn't all doom and gloom.

That evening, after I'd finished my apple crumble, a porter came to take me for my scan, which I assumed was going to be the ultrasound but no, strangely I ended up back in the CT scanner with a cannula hanging out of my arm connected to a machine that was going to flush me with a chemical contrast to help them investigate my blood vessels whilst scanning my chest. Luckily the radiographer told me in advance that it would give me a bit of a hot flush all over, together with the joyous sensation that I'd wet myself. I'm glad she warned me. As side effects go it was certainly one of the more novel ones.

Later that night, as I was about to try and get some sleep, a nurse came into my bay with yet more bad news. After reading the chest scan report it was apparent that I had several pulmonary emboli (PE) on my left lung. A PE is a type of clot in the blood vessels of the lung. This can be a life-threatening condition with the potential to cause respiratory or cardiac arrest, or even a stroke – should a portion of a clot break off and block a significant blood vessel. Whilst trying to remain calm on the outside I was freaking out on the inside. *"I have to give you this injection now"* she said firmly, an injection of an anti-coagulant drug to help break down the clots in my lung and stop new ones forming. As she injected me in my stomach she asked if I knew who referred me for the chest CT as there was no record of it in my notes. I didn't know. Somebody probably just forgot to sign it I thought. But apparently not – it became clear later that week that the chest scan had actually been ordered by mistake and hence the life-threatening clots had been discovered entirely by chance. In the space of two days I'd been diagnosed with two potentially life-threatening conditions. I didn't sleep much that night either, mostly worried about what they might find tomorrow.

During the next few days I had a second MRI scan together with an MRA, X-rays, ultrasound scans of my left leg and neck, as well as a range of other blood tests. It seemed if there was a test they could do, then they just threw me at it in a bid to see if anything stuck. However, by Friday with symptoms having cleared up and nothing to indicate any serious condition (other than the PE) I was discharged (after I'd had my dessert) and put on a course of Warfarin, another anti-coagulant drug, to lower my clotting risk for six months. I was relieved to get home; it had been a traumatic week. During my time in the hospital the staff were all fantastic. From the nurses (who were all amazed to hear about my ultramarathon exploits), to the doctors who scratched their heads trying to work out what was going on inside of me, to the nice lady that kept bringing me pudding. It was the NHS at its very finest. Back at home I had been signed off from work for a couple of weeks to recover. At least now I could get back to some level of normality and start running again. My feet were itching, although I'm not sure that wasn't the bed socks.

Whilst in hospital I had noticed that my left hip and lower back had started to ache a little but I didn't think much of it, putting it down to spending a week in bed. However when it started to worsen the following week it became more of a concern. With the pain getting worse every day, I made an appointment to see my GP to find out what was going on. At this point it had developed into a sharp pain in my lower back and left leg that was triggered by movement, only easing if I sat or lay still. The doctor's diagnosis was that a muscle spasm was compressing my sciatic nerve causing sciatica, which manifests itself with pain down one leg. *"It will ease in time"* was the medical advice topped off with some Co-Codamol for pain relief. A few days later and the pain was only worsening. Now I couldn't stand for more than a couple of minutes, nor could I walk very far without having to stop and sit down. Still thinking it was muscle related I paid a visit to Dave Adler, who after an examination agreed with the doctor. However with the pain still intensifying I went back to the GP who changed my prescription to Tramadol and

Diazepam for pain relief and as a muscle relaxant for the supposed spasm. Still the pain continued to get worse. I went back to see Dave a second time who this time had a deeper look and concluded it was most likely a problem with my back and not muscular at all. Back to the doctor I limped, now in severe pain, telling him what Dave had said. This time I saw a different GP, who examined my back and leg. *"I think you have a prolapsed disc that is causing the sciatica"* he told me, *"I will refer you for an MRI scan so we can see what is going on."* In the meantime in a further bid to ease the pain he prescribed me some oral Morphine solution to take on top of everything else, as well as Amitriptyline to help with the neurological pain of the sciatica.

Now with a sizeable handful of drugs being taken throughout the day, I was still in a lot of pain and could barely stand, let alone walk anywhere. It was a world away from the super fit individual who had ran sixty miles only weeks before. Far from turning out to be an invincible superhero I had become more akin to Mr Glass, the brittle comic-book loving supervillain played by Samuel L. Jackson in the film *Unbreakable*. To top things off, in the words of The Verve, *"the drugs don't work"*. They didn't exactly make things worse but they didn't appear to be doing a whole lot of good. So back to the GP I went yet again and was this time prescribed a higher dose of Morphine tablets that were longer lasting than the solution, together with Gabapentin, another drug to target the neuropathic pain. Finally with a mind-warping combination of medication I had started to see some relief, mostly because I was as high as a kite for most of the day. It was far from ideal but at least the pain was being managed. With my daily medication now being so strong I was unable to drive or even walk more than about eight-hundred metres, making me increasingly immobile and more reliant on others to ferry me around for even the most mundane of tasks.

After finding out the wait for an NHS MRI referral was likely to be in the region of eight weeks, I decided to pay and have the scan done privately to move things along. So after a bit of shopping around I had a referral made to the Cobalt Imaging Centre in Cheltenham and asked my sister give me a lift up there. Once I'd managed to get out of her low car without too much screaming I checked in with the receptionist and was shortly being slid into another MRI scanner. Unlike at the RUH I wasn't offered music to listen to during the scan. The radio in the changing room however was playing *Price Tag* by Jessie J which I thought was quite apt. If only it wasn't about the money. While my pain was now being better managed most of the time there were still certain positions that would cause me extreme discomfort, and lying still in a scanner for twenty minutes with my feet dangling over the end of the table turned out to be one of them. Knowing I had to remain as motionless as possible for the duration I bit down on my tongue and dug my nails into the palms of my hands in a bid to redirect my pain senses but the strength of the pain coming from my back and leg was far too great. After a couple of minutes I began to shake uncontrollably, much to the annoyance of the radiographer. *"Just another five minutes, do try to keep still"* he said through the otherwise quiet headphones. But five minutes or five seconds, I was already beyond it and had given up on trying to fight it. I was shaking and crying in pain all at the same time. Not a pretty sight for a grown man. With some luck – and the fact they did several scans – the images were clear enough to see what was going on and the consultant neuroradiologist diagnosed a prolapsed disc, bilateral spondylolysis and a degree of spondylolisthesis, all of which sounded pretty serious.

Spondylolysis is a defect of the vertebrae which can be caused by a hereditary condition; being born with a thin vertebral bone can make it more susceptible to fractures, but it can also be caused by repetitive trauma to the lumbar spine through sport. Spondylolysis is in turn the most common cause of spondylolisthesis – a slipping out of place of the vertebrae – although this can also be caused by a range of problems with the small joints in the back. It was a combination of these conditions that meant pressure was being applied to my sciatic nerve causing the all the pain.

Unfortunately, despite getting an MRI scan quicker, once I rejoined the realm of the NHS things slowed right down again. With the pain now largely under control, another appointment with my GP to go over the scan results ended up with a referral being made to the Spinal Assessment and Treatment Service (SATS) to determine how best to treat the problem.

It had now been just over ten weeks since I was first admitted to the RUH on my way to work that fateful Monday morning. In that time I had been through the medical mill and was still stuck within its outer workings. The morphine doses I had been taking had been high enough to mean I wasn't able to stay fully lucid. In fact, at the height of everything I would even fall asleep whilst talking, let alone know what I was talking about. I was like a narcoleptic Boris Johnson without the hair. It would take some weeks to wind the morphine dosage back down again to a level where I was still comfortable and able to return to work, let alone actually get treatment for the root cause of the pain. The referral to the SATS team saw me attend an outpatient clinic at Thornbury Hospital, which amazingly for any hospital in the 21st Century still had a free car park. Although I think the term 'hospital' was rather grand for it. If you ever find yourself going there, don't expect anything too special. The physiotherapist I saw looked at my MRI scans and read the report from Cobalt, before asking me for some background into my condition. He was a bit taken aback as I kept going into each avenue of detail and although I had a tendency to talk a lot, I tried to keep it brief but he still had a lot of typing to do. He then examined me and what became very clear very quickly was that there were a lot of positions I wasn't putting my left leg in, consciously or not. Whilst on a day-to-day basis the pain was being masked, as he was pulling, pushing and tweaking my leg around he was very successful at finding areas where the pain was hiding. What was clear was that the root of the problem was still present. His suggestion for treatment was to undergo a programme of physiotherapy, primarily to strengthen core muscles. Another option would be to consider a nerve block injection to temporarily block the leg and back pain but I couldn't have that while I remained on the Warfarin. Only as a final resort, if serious symptoms persisted, would surgery be considered as a treatment option. I was told that disc prolapses typically resolved themselves anywhere between six weeks and six months. I was certainly hoping for the former over the latter. However the treatment and recovery panned out it would need to be successful pretty quickly as I was already eating into my Chippenham Half Marathon training time.

The one question that has to be asked here is was the big weekend in any way to blame for my list of ailments? I asked this question to every health professional I saw along the way and nobody would commit to a firm yes. It was possible but there were no clear answers.

After a week in the hospital, none of the medical evidence pointed to or could confirm that I had suffered a stroke. Talking to my GP about it there was the theoretical possibility that part of a blood clot could have reached my brain and possibly caused a mini-stroke or TIA (transient ischaemic attack – a temporary disruption in the blood supply to part of the brain) but that was unproven and the case on it was closed. It could well have been some form of migraine, despite me having never suffered from them before. The blood clots on the lung were an incidental finding and were only small. It is possible that these could have been caused by the weekend, given that with aerobic fitness the number of red blood cells can increase essentially thickening the blood, hence giving rise to a higher clotting risk. Dehydration can also cause the blood to thicken in the same way. So it is possible I may have become dehydrated over the weekend which may have contributed to the problem. Finally the spine problems. Whilst it was feasible the slippage of the vertebrae could have in part been caused by the pounding out of extreme amounts of miles, it was equally possible that it was a long-standing condition that had been getting slowly worse with my advancing age. Prolapsed discs are commonplace and can be caused by anything from lifting heavy weights, to sneezing or bending over to pick something up off the floor. So it is possible that the run could have caused these problems although at the same time it could have been any number of things, nothing was clear or conclusive.

In short, did the big weekend break me? It was a possibility but not a certainty. Unless you count losing a couple of toenails, there was no conclusive medical evidence to prove anything. I guess it depends upon your opinion and perspective, although as a massive optimist I would naturally always veer towards probably not. Others might disagree. What it does make clear though is that even if you are as fit and healthy as you can be, you're still potentially never far from being incapacitated. That's just the way life is, which is why you need to make the most out of it and going forward that's certainly what I intended to do.

Given the turn of events since completing the big weekend it was pretty clear that me running a sub 1 hour 20 minutes race in September was going to be extremely unlikely, so Operation 119 could only sensibly be shelved for another day. At the start of June it was even in question whether I would even be running at all by September. Every health professional I had asked made it very clear to not run until the disc issue was resolved. How long was that going to take though? That was very far from being clear.

In my continual quest to dig for more answers, and never too shy to ask for a favour, I dropped an email to a doctor friend of mine, asking him if he knew anybody who could help shed any further light on the problem. As luck would have it he did know one person who fitted the bill perfectly. A person amongst whose specialist skills were assessment, diagnosis and treatment planning for patients suffering from problems of the lower back. He sounded ideal. However despite everybody involved being keen, all attempts to try and get a referral through the system failed, as unfortunately they circumvented the process. But favours trump red tape and a few emails later, I had arranged an unofficial appointment for a consultation during his lunch hour. Result.

After listening intently to my now protracted recent medical history and reviewing the MRI scans, I was sent for x-rays of my spine. Of particular interest to see was a weight-bearing x-ray which very plainly showed the spondylolisthesis. It was clear to see the vertebrae in question had slipped out from the one above, by 10mm – a slippage of 20%. This is categorised as a grade one slippage, which is the least serious of classifications. After reviewing the x-rays his opinion was that as long as I remained pain free I should be able to return to running. If however the spondylolisthesis deteriorated further and the pain returned, then treatment for the problem may be required. As such I was given an open appointment to come back at any time. A letter was then written to my GP, reverse engineering me back into the system. Overall it was a positive result and things were starting to improve.

By this time my pain was receding and I was slowly winding back the amount of medication I was taking. As frustrating as it was to still be taking it all, I couldn't just suddenly stop popping the pills, and my GP had given me an eight-week schedule to reduce the morphine and other drugs. Being such an optimist though I figured things were going well enough for me to start dropping it all quicker. I was feeling good, and certainly keen to get off the drugs, so I came up with my own (slightly faster) reduction plan. Initially everything seemed to be going fine, right up until the day I decided to take a slow walk to the gym, which was about a mile from my house.

The initial quarter of a mile was fine but then as I walked I began to feel increasingly weak. Within the span of a minute I went from feeling normal to being absolutely exhausted. My legs suddenly felt as if they were going to collapse beneath me, and feeling anxious I quickly made my way to the nearest wall and sat down. As I sat there wondering what to do next I began to shake uncontrollably. What was happening to me? I waited a few minutes to see if the sensation would pass, but after it didn't and with the anxiety only increasing I made the strategic decision to call my wife to come and rescue me. Back at home I managed to call my GP who told me I was almost certainly suffering from morphine withdrawal, and the solution was simple – stop trying to wind down the dosage so quickly. Apparently I wasn't superhuman and immune from the effects of morphine dependency. Back to the slow plan.

As I was cleared for a tentative return to running, a week later I successfully made it to the gym and managed to run for two miles on a treadmill. It was a cautious affair but after having spent months barely able to even walk it was a positively glorious experience. I was quite naturally nervous at even the prospect of running again after everything that had happened and I fully expecting to not make it past a few steps before being forced to stop. Luckily though that wasn't the case. I kept the speed slow and the distance short. I didn't have anything to prove to anyone. I just wanted to see if I still worked, and I did. The journey to recovery had begun.

After fourteen weeks off I was finally well enough to return to work and some semblance of normality. A couple of weeks later I eased back into spending my lunchtimes running, with a short three-mile run with Bear taking in a short loop up and around one of the smaller hills we had conquered the previous winter. This time around however it nearly destroyed me. We didn't run fast, and certainly didn't run far, but by the time we got back to the office my legs were actually shaking – and this time not from morphine withdrawal. Clearly three months doing no exercise at all had somewhat negatively affected my fitness levels. Getting back to where I had been before the troubles was obviously going to take some effort.

By now the summer was in full swing and as we came into the start of July with the Chippenham Half Marathon only ten weeks away, I was still only running a couple of miles a few times a week. My goal of running a personal best was looking pretty shaky – even with my optimistic perspective – although I was determined to push on and run the race anyway. Because I knew I wasn't going to be running anything particularly fast I took my time easing back into training, making each step up carefully and not going too far or too fast. As the weeks passed I slowly incremented my mileage, picking up the speed a touch as I went. I went from four-mile runs, to five, then six, then eight, building the distance up slowly. However, whilst my fitness had been improving, my confidence needed a bit of a high-mileage speed boost.

With just two weeks to go until the race I asked Phil if he fancied a ten-mile run to see if I could gauge what pace I should race at. The plan was initially to try and run somewhere between eight-thirty and nine minutes per mile, which I thought at the time I said it was still highly ambitious. Setting out on a warm August morning we pushed the first couple of miles and still feeling good kept pushing all the way around, eventually completing the run in just over an eight minute average. By the time we stopped I was shattered and could barely stand but I was pleased. It was exactly the boost I needed.

Race day came around and standing on the start line in Chippenham I was pleased to just be there. After how events had unfolded following the big weekend, running at all was a bonus, but to actually be back in the position where I could confidently run a race and expect to finish in a reasonable time was fantastic.

Keeping my head down at the start and letting everyone else

run their own race, I managed to keep a steady pace throughout and finish in a respectable 1 hour 47 minutes. I was back. I might have been much further down the fitness ladder than where I fell off some months before but I was climbing and knew I would get back to the levels I had previously achieved.

With Chippenham over and dusted it was time to look forward to 2014 and what to do next. During a summer holiday to Scotland in July I went on a boat trip around Loch Lomond where I was entranced by the incredible scenery. The landscape was beautiful and I thought how great it would be to run around it. After I got back home I did a bit of research and found out about a race called the Hoka Highland Fling, which is a fifty-three mile ultramarathon that runs up the West Highland Way footpath from Glasgow at the end of April. I was sold and after some discussion, I also managed to convince Bear that it was a good enough idea that we entered. After all it's not such a big jump from forty-six miles to fifty-three. Is it? Ask me in May.

What this whole process has taught me more than anything else is that through tenacity and hard work it really is possible to achieve seemingly superhuman feats. We can't all be as slim or as fit as the elite, guys like Dean Karnazes, but actually that doesn't matter. What matters is that you set yourself challenging goals and work hard at making them happen. It's not about natural ability or luck, it's about hard work and determination. The sense of satisfaction from seeing the effort you have invested in something manifest itself into reality is extremely rewarding.

The thing to remember is that sometimes the goals you set yourself can, on the face of it, seem a little tough, but they are the fun ones. That's when it pays to be a delusional optimist.

Epilogue

On Thursday 30th May 2013, three months after completing a challenge inspired by the tragic diagnosis of my friend Remo Del-Greco, I received news informing me that he had lost his battle with cancer – just one month and three days after his fifty-ninth birthday. Whilst not entirely unexpected, having spent the last few weeks in a hospice, it was very sad news that stopped me in my tracks. I sat down and sobbed at the loss of a good man. He was quite simply one of the nicest people I have ever had the pleasure to meet. He was funny, smart and genuine. Here was a man who despite knowing he was in the closing days of his life, still made sure he sent me a get well soon card when he heard that I was unwell. I was touched beyond words to receive the card. Proof if any were ever needed of the heart of this man. His passing has left a large hole for everyone who knew him, especially his wife Yvonne and five children, Donna, Paolo, Joseph, James and Sam. I consider myself lucky to have met such a brave man, who in the face of terrible adversity simply played it down and remained stoic to the end. As somebody who has a fear of death he has been inspirational to me and I'm pleased that I had the opportunity to tell him as much. He knew that he was my inspiration to undertake the challenges that make up this book and I'm pleased that he was around to see a successful outcome and the money it raised for good causes. Rest well Remo, you will be missed. As my mum always told me, *"life's not fair"*.

Acknowledgements

Whilst writing is itself a solitary process, putting together something like this can only be done with help and support coming from many corners. This book and indeed the story that it contains, was only made possible with thanks to a great number of people. In recognition of that fact I would like to thank each and every one of them for helping me turn an idea into a reality.

Firstly I would like to say a special thank you to both Phil Westlake and Bill Graham for their continual support over the years. Without either of them, none of this would ever have happened in the first place. Whether it has been out running, coaching, or just talking things through both of these guys have helped bring out the best in my running, giving me the encouragement I sometimes needed. I would also like to especially thank Bear (Rudi Schlenker) and Guy Lucas for being insane enough to undertake the very same challenges I did and keep me company on many long, cold and wet runs listening to me talk far too much, spouting plenty of rubbish and putting the world to rights. You certainly learn a lot about people when you spend many hours running in their company and I'm pleased to say it was all positive.

A large number of other friends and runners played an instrumental part in helping me train and stay inspired and motivated through the winter of 2012/13. There are too many to name individually (plus I would hate to offend anyone by leaving them out), so suffice to say thank you all for accompanying me on so many runs in the cold and the wet and giving me friendly faces to run with. Lunchtimes; weekends; and early mornings alike, it almost made all the hard work fun.

A very special thank you has to go to all the amazing staff at the Royal United Hospital in Bath, in particular those on the Acute Stroke Unit, who looked after me so well when things looked a bit grim. They really did represent the NHS at its very best. Thank you for taking care of me. I am also incredibly appreciative of my own GP Dr Richard Berkeley for being so patient with me and my constant questioning at every appointment. Thanks to David Adler too for helping keep me running with his physiotherapy magic when I needed it and to Jonathan Robinson and the Human Performance Centre team at the University of Bath who helped point my training in the right direction and also answered so many inane questions about how it all works.

I would like to show my appreciation to Macmillan Cancer Support for giving me one of their bond places for the Bath Half Marathon at such short notice, as well as everyone who donated so very generously to my begging, particularly the members of the RF Owners Club and the committee of Bitton Road Runners who all gave wedges of cash in hard times.

For all the people who read snippets of this book as I wrote it and drip fed it to them (primarily Bear Schlenker, Phil Westlake and Andy Hulcoop), I am indebted to you for the invaluable feedback that helped spot the typos, contribute ideas and shape it into the story it ended up being. Likewise, without the amazing help and support of Richard Jones at Tangent Books, you wouldn't even be holding this book now. I would also like to especially thank Neil Kerfoot for casting his medical eye over my hazy recollections of numerous ailments for accuracy.

Finally, but of course undeniably the biggest and most important thank you must go to my wife and family who over the years have constantly tolerated all my harebrained schemes and continue to give me both the support and freedom to be the person I am at heart.

Additional Information

For more information on me and the book, including photos, GPS data and various other odds and sods, or even just if you want to get in touch, why not catch up with me somewhere online.

Twitter: @IraRainey

Blog: http://www.notbionic.co.uk

Facebook: http://www.facebook.com/fm2gm

The Green Man Ultra is organised by Ultra Running. They organise lots of other ultramarathons all around the UK.

http://www.ultrarunning.uk.com/

More information about the Bristol Community Forest Path and the Green Man Challenge can be found on the Closer to the Countryside website.

http://www.closertothecountryside.co.uk/

Bitton Road Runners is a running club based in the east of Bristol which caters for all running abilities. Founded in 1986 to help people better enjoy the sport of running, they are a thriving club with both junior and senior sections. New members are always welcome.

http://www.bittonroadrunners.co.uk/

We are all affected by cancer, so why not donate the money you would normally spend from just one night in a month to help somebody else instead? Macmillan Cancer Support provide practical, medical, emotional and even financial support to people suffering from cancer and those who care for them, but they can only continue this work with the generosity of people like you.

http://www.macmillan.org.uk/